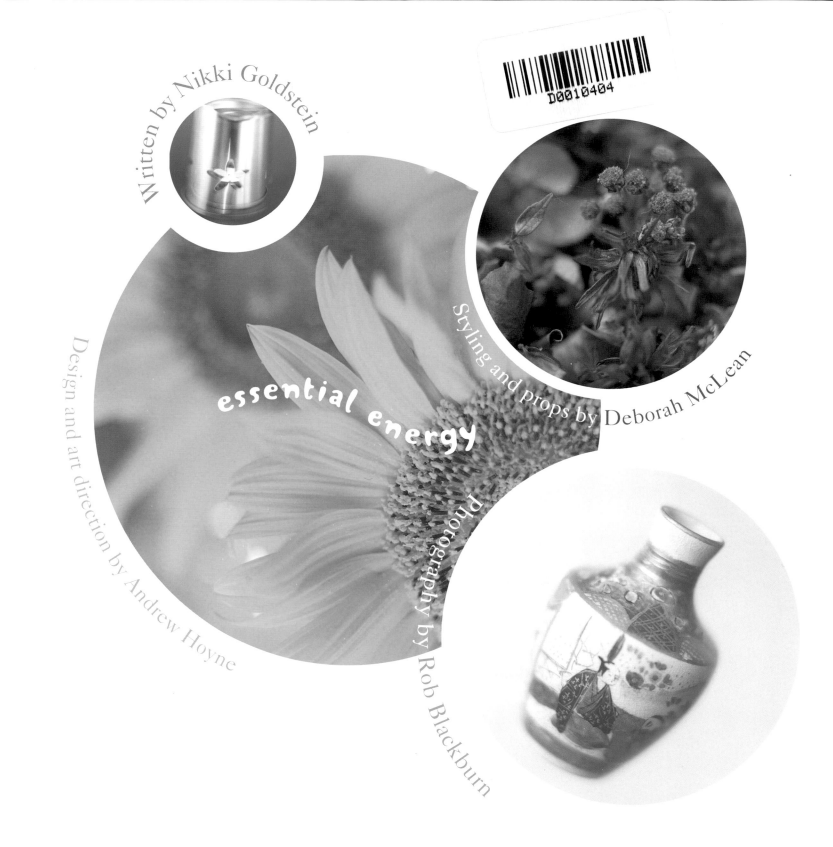

Written by Nikki Goldstein

Styling and props by Deborah McLean

essential energy

Design and art direction by Andrew Hoyne

Photography by Rob Blackburn

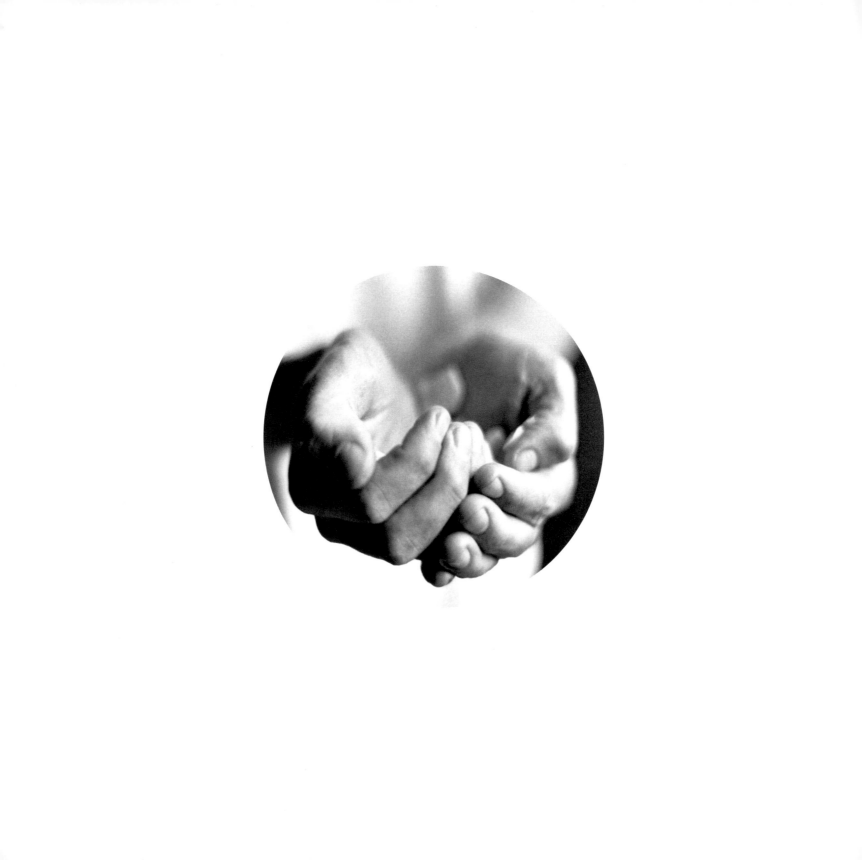

contents

in the

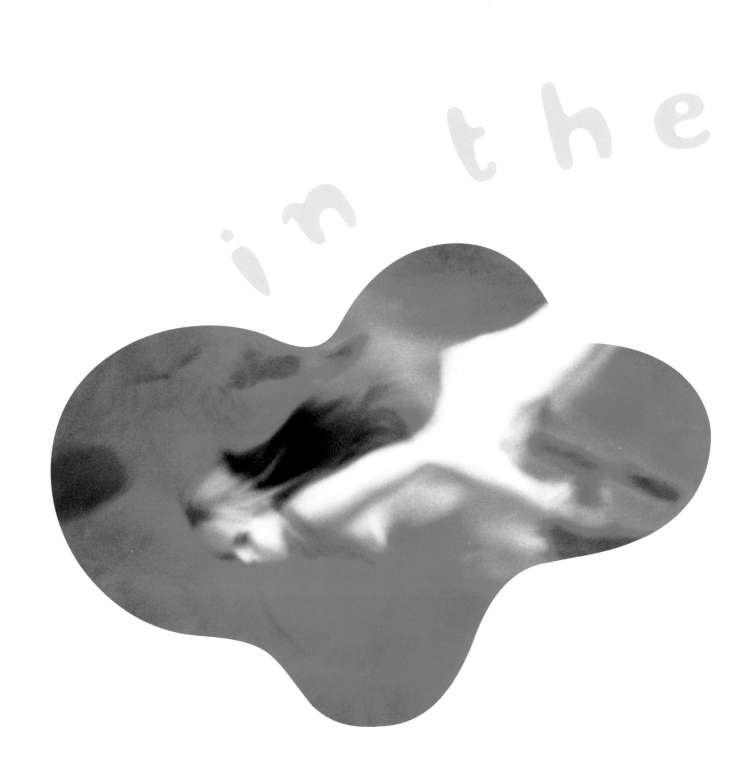

the discovery of nature's fragrant pharmacopoeia

The roots of aromatherapy lie in the history of botanical medicine: For many thousands of years, plants and flowers have been used to heal humans. Plant essences played a significant role in the healing disciplines and cosmetic lore of ancient Egypt, China, Greece, Rome, and India—where in many instances they are still used today. Essential oils found their way into incense and ointments, perfumes and potions used to beautify the body, heal all ills, and satisfy the hedonistic and demanding gods. The word "perfume" comes from two Latin words, *per* meaning "through" and *fumum* meaning "smoke," signifying the origin of all perfumery—incense. But aromatherapy as we know it today, as a comprehensive physical, psychological, metaphysical, and cosmetic science, was transformed by a pioneering French chemist, René-Maurice Gattefossé, as recently as the early twentieth century.

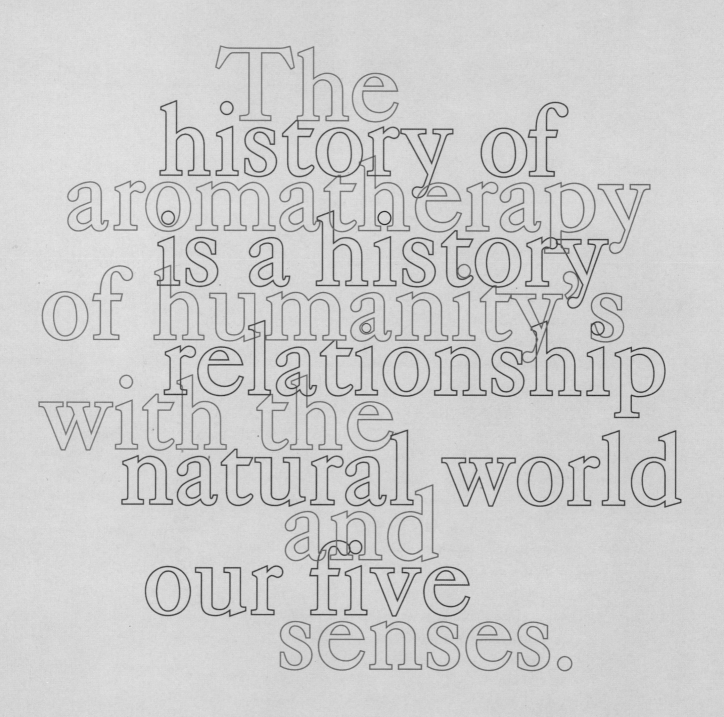

The history of aromatherapy is a history, of humanity's relationship with the natural world and our five senses.

Modern research is confirming Gattefossé's original suspicions of its benefits to humankind, but the early practice of aromatherapy was largely an anecdotal science. It relied on the spoken word, and many thousands of years of trial and error. Yet, this circumstantial evidence is not imprecise. One imagines that with a grunt and a simple gesture, primitive humans communicated which plant would heal a wounded leg and which herb could cure a fever. Over time such knowledge became sacred and revered. The use of this natural pharmacopoeia seems unscientific by the modern methods of studying empirical data, but we know from history that aromatherapy, or at least the science of treatment with essential oils, played a significant role through the ages of humankind.

The history of aromatherapy

Aromatherapy is the art and science of treating human illness with essential oils. These volatile essences of plants and flowers have been used for healing for many thousands of years, allied with touch, taste, and smell. The history of aromatherapy is a history of humanity's relationship with the natural world and our own five senses.

Prehistory

Aromatic cues ensured the safety and well-being of entire communities because memory came in the form of odor, not words. Early females used smell to determine a man's state of health,

his status among his male counterparts, and what kind of food he was eating. And it was smell that alerted tribal members to the hungry tiger at the mouth of the cave. Pricked by the sharp scent of death hovering with the dawn of each day, the olfactory ability was awakened.

By relying on their sense of smell to survive, early humans learned to recognize the various scents nature provided—animals, plants, flowers, trees, grains, roots, and resins. This system of classification led them to discover the tremendous relationship between odor and flavor. Condiments, spices, and herbs—whose medicinal properties they later discovered—extended their olfactory repertoire. To broaden their diet, they extracted oil from oleaginous grains, and through experimentation they discovered how to use oils to protect their skin and treat their hair. The enjoyment of food gave rise to the idea that fragrance was pleasurable, sexual, and even spiritual. Before they knew how to make fire, humans had learned that heat transformed the odors and flavors of vegetables and flesh. The first religious practices were born out of the concept that fire would convey their devotion to the gods in the sky, via coils of rising scent.

The discovery of fire and all the progress it brought— pottery, among other skills—led to the construction of the first distillation equipment. The remains of a still found recently in Mesopotamia are said to be over 5,000 years old. Initial uses for these devices were probably of a culinary nature, but it is likely that aromatic oils were also discovered around this time.

Egypt

The Egyptians were the first true aromatherapists. Fragrance was an integral part of Egyptian life, permeating both secular and spiritual aspects. The early aromatherapists were priests, who administered scented ointments to worshipers as part of elaborate religious rituals. In Heliopolis, the city devoted to the sun god Ra, incense was burned three times a day. Incense was always burned at the opening of a shrine, at the coronation of a pharaoh, and all national celebrations. The souls of the dead were thought to ascend as a cloud of smoke. The amazingly complex perfume for the gods, Kyphi, was a sophisticated cocktail of essential oils: peppermint, saffron, juniper, acacia, and henna, all mixed with wine and honey, resin, myrrh, and raisins. The concoction was mixed and made into a paste and allowed to solidify. It was then ready to be placed into a burner as an offering.

Probably the first aromatic practice dedicated specifically to healing was fumigation. Plant oils were burned until smoke engulfed a sickroom thereby combating evil spirits and banishing them from an ailing body. Although the Egyptians could not identify the powerful antibacterial, antifungal, and antiviral properties of the plants, the effect produced a cleansing of the atmosphere and subsequent purification of the lungs.

The Egyptian penchant for incense is well recorded. In fact, military campaigns were mounted to ensure a stable supply of the prized cedar, which all but bankrupted the indigenous cedar forests of Lebanon. Queen Hatshepsut of the New Kingdom (1558–1085 B.C.) put incense on the cultural map. She was the Queen Victoria of the ancient world and her voracious appetite for power and sovereignty took her to Punt (or Pwenet), somewhere in Somalia, to capture the precious gum resins needed for domestic and religious incense. Her expedition is recorded for posterity on the walls of her temple at Deir al-Bahari near Thebes. This powerful ruler, who had herself immortalized in the headdress of a king and the mane of a lion, had a botanical garden created on the ramps of the temple. The plants came from Punt and she boasted: "I have led them on water and on land to explore the waters of inaccessible channels, and I have reached the incense trees." It was the journey into the next world that preoccupied Egyptians most. And to this end they went to great lengths to ensure the dead a swift and comfortable journey to what awaited them. Aromatics in beautiful alabaster jars and ebony coffers contained ointments they believed would render the skin of the deceased supple after his arrival in the next world. The embalming process involved eviscerating the body, which was washed in salt, and

> "Egyptians wore scented cones of animal fat impregnated with essential oils from the land of Punt (modern Somalia).
> Before the distillation of alcohol, fatty oils from plant or animal sources were the first solvents for perfumes."
>
> *Fragrance: The Story of Perfume from Cleopatra to Chanel*

filling the cavities with myrrh and oakmoss. The oakmoss, which was imported from Greece, had an exquisite, soft, sweet scent that was incredibly tenacious. It contained usnic acid, an antibiotic that performed well in the mummifying process. Pine resin, another essential oil with antimicrobial properties, was also included in this careful ritual to send the body into eternity. As the Egyptian civilization progressed, the human body became an object of great admiration, deserving of the most elaborate pampering with perfumed oils and cosmetics. Initially, many of the cosmetics were used for magical purposes—worn as amulets to ward off hexes and curses set upon them by jealous gods and unsympathetic energies.

Thick mascara was painted on the eyelids and lashes and used to protect the eyes from the harsh sun. Many of the creams and lotions were used for medicinal reasons or as anti-aging remedies. Almost all the cosmetics bore a scent: African frankincense and myrrh, lily, pine, cedar of Lebanon, bitter almond, mint, and other herbs. These aromatics were used to scent a base of vegetable oil or animal fats. The priests would soak fruits and herbs in the base and prepare ointments and fragrance cones to be worn under wigs and massaged into the skin. The Egyptians employed the use of essential oils in daily baths and massage and understood the benefits to the skin and nervous system. But it took many thousands of years of civilization for Europeans to recognize the therapeutic and preventive value of Egyptian beautification rituals.

In his book *Fragrance: The Story of Perfume from Cleopatra to Chanel*, Edwin T. Morris explains that cosmetics, creams, and pomades were very early vehicles for scent. The fats, oils, and waxes of cosmetics were the first carriers of essential oils and wereconsidered scented products. A stick perfume, for example, is an essential oil dissolved in solid wax. Even today's lipsticks are perfume products with dyes added.

Candles, blended with essential oils, are fragranced homewares—descendants of the scent-releasing lamp, one of the world's most ancient artifacts.

Israel

No study of aromatherapy is complete without reference to the Bible and no passage is more celebratory of scent than the Song of Songs (below). Each stanza is infused with the intoxication of scent intimately shared by two lovers in an exotic garden. In all cultures, scent and spirit have been linked. The passage is said to be an allegory of the relationship between the material and the divine.

She: While the king rests on his bed,
my perfume gives off its fragrance.
My lover is like a bag of myrrh
lying between my breasts.
My beloved is like a cluster of henna
plucked from the vineyards of Ein Gedi.

He: My love among the young women is like
a lily among thistles.

She: My love among the young men is like an
apple tree among the trees of the forest.
I long to sit in his shade and to taste his sweet fruit
on my palate.

He: Your lips drip honey, my bride.
Honey and milk lie under your tongue, and the
fragrance of your dress is the fragrance of Lebanon.
A closed garden is my sister, my bride.
A closed well

A sealed fountain.
Your plants form an orchard of pomegranates,
laden with ripe fruit and sweet spices — henna and
nard, nard and saffron, calamus and cinnamon,
branches of incense, myrrh, aloes
—all the sweetest spices.
The well in your garden is a fountain of living
waters rushing down from Lebanon.

She: O north wind, awake.
South wind, rise up.
Blow on my garden and let my spices flow.
Let my love enter his garden and eat his sweet fruit.

He: My sister, my bride,
I have entered my garden.
I have gathered my myrrh with my spices.
I have eaten my honeycomb with my honey.
I have drunk my wine with my milk.
Eat, friends, drink!
And become drunk with love!

Extracted passages (not necessarily in order) from Diane Wolkstein's *First Love Stories*, translated from the Hebrew version that modern secular scholars consider to be a compilation of texts composed at various times between 900 and 300 B.C. Orthodox Jews and Christians believe the poem to be divinely inspired. Legend has it that the poem referred to King Solomon and his love affair with the Queen of Sheba.

At the time the Song of Songs was composed (some hundred years before the birth of Christ), frankincense and myrrh had reached the Mediterranean cultures. Saffron, while no longer used as a perfume ingredient today, comes from the Arabic *zafran*, meaning "yellow"; the stamens of this flower were used not only for aroma but for color. Aloes were probably aloewood, an Indian product that was exported to Asia at that time. Aloewood is distilled today to extract its deliciously sweet essence, which is much prized in East Asia. The nard or "spikenard" was another Indian ingredient, which according to the Bible was used by Mary Magdalene to perfume the feet of Jesus. It is still used by Indian women today to perfume their hair. Perfume is referred to in the Bible story of Judith, who used it as a means to seduce Holofernes and kill him. We also find that myrtle was used at the original Feast of the Tabernacles, while olive branches and pine boughs were used in the festivals observed after the return of the exiles from Babylon. One of the promises to Israel reads, "instead of the brier shall come the myrtle tree." The Hebrew word for myrtle is *hadas*, which was linked to Hadassah, the Hebrew name for Queen Esther.

Greece

While the Egyptians initiated the art of extracting essences from plants by heating them in clay containers, it was the Greek alchemists who invented distillation two centuries later. By the seventh century B.C., Athens and Corinth enjoyed a flourishing business making perfumed products that were contained in magnificent vessels. Olive oil, almond oil, castor oil, sesame oil, and linseed oil were used as the carriers for perfumes scented with lily, marjoram, thyme, sage, rose, anise, and iris root. Scents were widely used by both men and women and the burning of incense on municipal altars became commonplace. The first treatise on scent, in fact the first text on aromatherapy, was the inventory written by the botanist Theophrastus entitled "Concerning Odors." He listed all Greek and imported aromatics and discussed ways in which they could be most elegantly blended by a perfumer. This diligent scientist considered the properties of the various oils used as carriers of scent, scents in wine, the use of dried flowers and herbs, the shelf life of scented products, the suitability of various scents for certain states of mind, and the use of scent for the respective health of both sexes. Theophrastus also explored the process by which we are able to perceive smells and noted the similarity between smell and taste.

Dioscorides, a Greek physician, noted that dranculus, a plant with a stalk "spotted like a serpent's belly," keeps cancer in check, is an abortifacient, cures gangrene, and is good for eyesight. Galen, another Greek physician, who was one of the world's most celebrated herbalists, wrote a text that remained the standard botanical reference right through to the Middle Ages. He provided a recipe from a combination of 150 plants, animal parts, minerals, and even precious stones. A panacea for ills from headaches to leprosy, theriac was still prescribed in France until the seventeenth century, and was carried aboard seagoing vessels for hundreds of years. Alexander the Great used aromatics with great abandon and his own funeral pyre was a lavish display of sight and smell, burning costly resins that hung in the air like a great fragrant bird circling the body. Cleopatra (69–30 B.C.), was the last and most famous monarch of the dynasties established by Alexander in the East. Cleopatra was a young Greek woman who presided over the final moments of greatness of the kingdom of Egypt. She needed the might of imperial Rome to support her control of the throne of Egypt, and in return Rome used the wealth of Egypt to pay its legions. Cleopatra and her brother were the children of a Macedonian general who bribed his way to the throne of Egypt after the death of Alexander the Great. The two children were married, in the custom of the pharaohs, but split as their aspirations for power grew.

An appeal to Julius Caesar, the executor of the father's will, brought him to Alexandria, where Cleopatra seduced him. There are no prizes for guessing who won what battle. According to history, Cleopatra was no great beauty, although she was striking and seductive. She used perfume and cosmetics to her advantage and wore all the adornments of the day—henna in her hair, rouge on her cheeks, hands, and buttocks, and Kyphi in strategic places. Cleopatra knew how to use the magical art of scent to seduce and control. When she received the Roman General Mark Antony on her royal barge, she had the sails scented with exotic perfume, incense burners surrounded her throne, and her lithe body was clothed in diaphanous robes that were scented with the finest aromatics Egypt could produce. Antony was captivated and left all sense behind—except perhaps that of smell. Cleopatra was learned in all the healing arts and was as masterful with poison as she was with perfume. There are many reports of experiments on condemned prisoners with lethal agents that brought on spasms and death. On her last night in the mortal world, before she devoured the poisoned fig that killed her, she bathed and had herself massaged from head to toe in the finest fragrances. When the Roman soldiers broke into her chamber, they found her dead, but even in death her scent was seductive and divine, befitting her royal status.

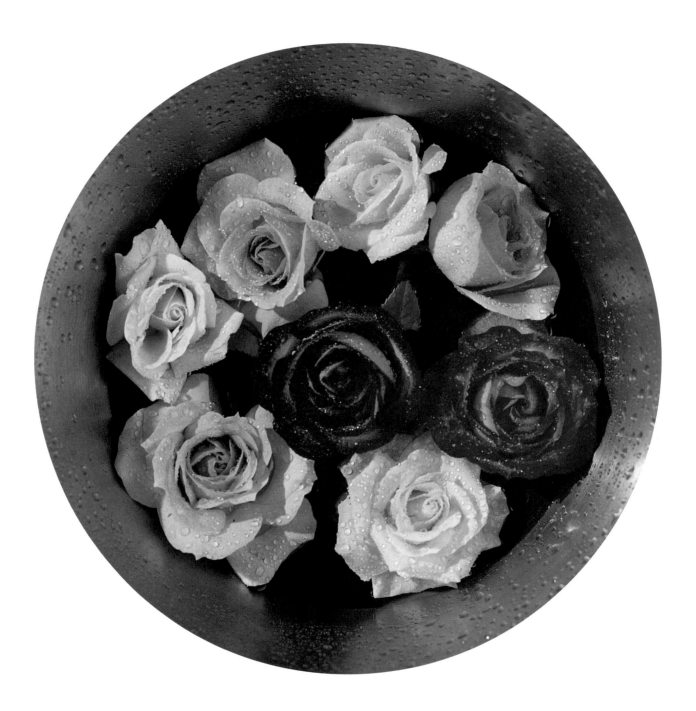

Rome

Rome borrowed much from Greek culture; however, it was the hedonistic Romans who spread the use of aromatics far and wide. People literally bathed in perfume. Slaves known as cosmetae prepared scents for Roman women, who used pigeon droppings to lighten their hair and lead to bleach their skin. Many thousands of tons of frankincense and myrrh were imported from southern Arabia.

The indulgent Emperor Nero built the first air-conditioning system, which delivered the intoxicating scent of roses throughout the palace via an elaborate system of silver pipes.

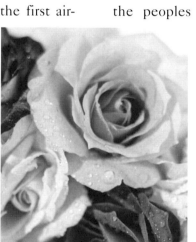

In one famous episode a guest was asphyxiated by showers of rose-scented water. The Romans prized the rose above all other flowers. They adorned themselves with roses at feasts and festivals, decorated their villas with flowering branches, and on the occasion of military victory had the streets lined with petals. Nero used four million sesterces of roses (hundreds of thousands of dollars' worth) for one celebration, and the feast of the Rosalia was created to honor this flower.

By A.D. 3, Rome had become the bathing capital of the world. More than a thousand fragrant watering holes were located throughout the city and all were scented with the *buccheri*, ointments held in red clay containers. Each bath had its own *unctuarium* where bathers were oiled and massaged.

Conquests, crusades, and the growth of trade helped to spread the knowledge and techniques of herbalists and perfumers. Alexander's conquest of Afghanistan resulted in the marriage of Greek and Indian medicinal lore. The Romans' great trade routes enabled them to import East Indian spices and gum resins from Arabia, where some important new aromatic products and processes were being developed. By the second century A.D., Alexandria was the meeting-ground for all the peoples of the ancient world—Egyptians, Romans, Greeks, Jews, Syrians, and Persians. And while the Roman religion and culture began to decline, other religions and theories began to grow—Christianity, Gnosticism, and the practice of alchemy. The alchemists among these cultures believed the spark of divinity could be found in matter. By submitting mineral and botanical substances to intense heat in alembics, stills, and baths, they hoped to separate the divine spirit hiding in the banal. The essential oil extracted from a mixture of water and plant matter was a by-product of their experiments.

In the beginning, perfume oils were almost always the result of the distillation of plant material with water, but eventually alcohol could be extracted from the still. From the testing grounds of Alexandria a tradition of alchemists perpetuated the master's art—right through the Christian and Byzantine periods.

The Arab world

Byzantium was a thriving center of knowledge and culture during the Dark Ages in Europe. Islam was the link between antiquity and the modern world, and Byzantium the place through which the vast learning of the Greco-Roman world was filtered across Asia, North Africa, and southern Europe. The writings of great alchemists, botanists, and philosophers, translated from Greek and Latin, were to fuel the work of Islamic alchemists. Ar-Razi (c.850–c.924) was a famous herbalist and physician of Baghdad and Jabir ibn Hayyan, or Gerber, wrote an encyclopedia of all knowledge, the *Summa Perfectionis*. Yakub al-Kindi left a work entitled *The Book of Perfume Chemistry and Distillation*, in which he explained the distillation of musk and the balsams. He also described the manufacture of attar of rose. Ibn-Sina (980–1037) was a philosopher whose experimental works gained him the name "Prince of Pharmacists." Attar of rose was his cure for the diseases of the digestive tract.

In addition to the establishment of a great body of literature, Arab scientists made practical improvements to the techniques of distillation. Measurement became important and pharmacy became known as the art of *mizan*, the scales. The Arabs introduced filtration in laboratory experiments, borrowed from Asian scientists who had entered the Islamic sphere. Experiments were carried out with inorganic compounds, including petroleum extracts, and the Arabs mastered glassmaking, which meant they could manufacture vessels able to withstand the heat of distillation. Another leap forward was the invention of true soapmaking. By the eighth century in Syria, the Arabs had learned to put water through a mixture of wood ash and quicklime—the first manufacture of solid soap, which would be scented with aromatics.

The Arabs established extensive trade routes that linked India, China, the Mediterranean, and Indonesia with the Arab world. The benefits of this new trade system were many. The Hindu numerical system replaced the old Roman tables, the use of paper and paper money became commonplace, and the wide use of the compass—an old Chinese invention—changed the navigational abilities of the Arab fleets.

Spice became one of the principal commodities of the time. Spices were also considered drugs and were worth as much as the most precious jewels. Edwin T. Morris reveals a document by Amr ibn-Bahr (864 or 869) of Basra, who lists incense from Yemen, balsam from Egypt, saffron and flavored syrups from Isfahan, sumin from Kirman, jasmine ointment from Fars, sandalwood from India, and cassia from China. Scented gloves were valuable goods and sugar was sold as a precious commodity as well as syrups scented with rose and violet. Gum mastic was imported from Chios in the Aegean Islands, ambergris and civet from Ethiopia, agarwood from India and Burma, and ginger, cinnamon, clove, and nutmeg from the East Indies. Musk came from Szechwan or Tibet and camphor came from western China or the coastal cities of Hangchou and Canton.

Of all the aromatics in the Arabic repertoire the rose was most highly prized. The Sufis encouraged the practice of meditation in a rose garden, which is still one of the most common motifs in Persian carpets and miniatures. The rose was the symbol of the highest spiritual attainment and was supposed to transport the essence of Allah on its fragrance. A Turkish merchant introduced the cult of the rose into the Ottoman Empire, which became the world's largest rose plantation. The damask rose is the last remnant of the Arab culture in that part of the world. Islam played a leading role in the development of aromatic healing. Without the Arabs, the knowledge of Greece and Rome may have been lost forever. Through their endeavors, an advanced level of chemical and pharmaceutical technology thrived and made a variety of goods available to the entire civilized world. The Arabs perfected the still, which has had an incalculable influence on fragrance and flavor. Distillation of essential oils of fruits, flowers, and vegetable substances has provided one of the most sophisticated paths to pleasure known to mankind.

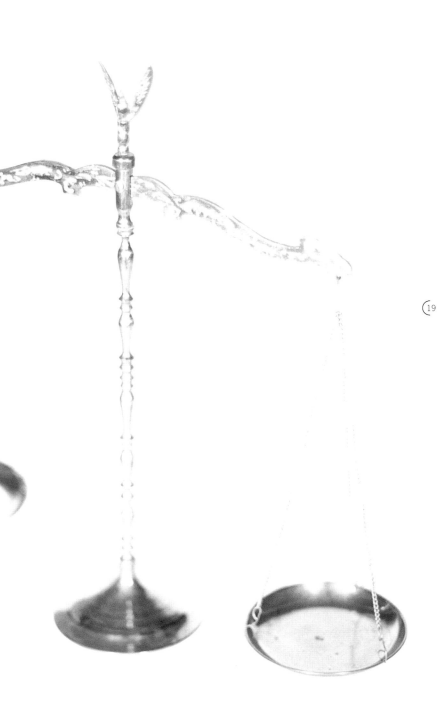

India

India was the fragrant garden of the world, boasting a wealth of aromatic plants that stretched from the Himalayas to the warm waters of the Indian Ocean. The Indians relished the use of fragrant balms in the rituals of bathing and the art of seduction. This extract from the *Kamasutra* (A.D. 400) details the role of aromatic plants in daily life. A regular high caste Hindu male must: get up early in the morning, answer the call of nature, wash his teeth, smear his body with just a little fragrant paste, inhale fragrant smoke, wear a flower, give the lips a rub with wax and red juice, look at his face in the mirror, chew betel leaves along with some mouth deodorants, and then attend to his work. The women of India, unfettered by the conservative conventions of Islam, adorned their bodies with jewels, scanty veils, and fragrance. The Buddhists, Jains, and Brahmans all publicized the benefits of frequent bathing and encouraged the use of fragrant pastes, oils, and powders.

The Indians scented screens, fans, mats, and clothes with vetiver and sandalwood. To cover the stench of cremation, they burned sandalwood and other spices with the bodies. Buddhists described the journey to the afterlife as the passage to the "fragrant mountain." During the spring festivals, colored and scented waters were sprayed through the air, dousing merrymakers in rich, lasting scents. Edwin T. Morris discovered one early author, Gangadhara, who wrote: "This science of cosmetics and perfumery is helpful in the worship of gods, which requires the use of auspicious perfumes and incense; it contributes to the pleasures of men; it leads to the attainment of the three ends of human life (religious merit, worldly prosperity, and sensual enjoyment); it removes one's own poverty; it contributes to the pleasures of kings and it gives the highest delight to the minds of accomplished ladies."

The Indian perfumer was an important person in civic life. He mixed and macerated fragrant piles of spice, chips of sandalwood, bright crystals of benzoin, roots and leaves, petals and stems into oils, cosmetics, pastes, and incense. Jasmine and sesame oil were mixed to make "Chameli ka tel," a pomade used to dress hair. The long, sleek midnight locks would retain the scent and the tresses would benefit from the oil—rendering hair glossy and silky and promoting a healthy scalp. The use of aromatics permeated every facet of Indian culture. One potent example is the use of the *abhyanga* or fragrant massage (still used in India today). Not only used by humans, this technique was employed as a seduction tool to encourage the mating of male and female elephants. After her bath, the female was covered in fragrance to excite the bull. The list of Indian aromatics is vast. Sandalwood, patchouli, vetiver, spikenard, gum benzoin, agarwood, jasmine, and rose were all found in abundance and were used for medicinal and religious purposes for centuries.

20

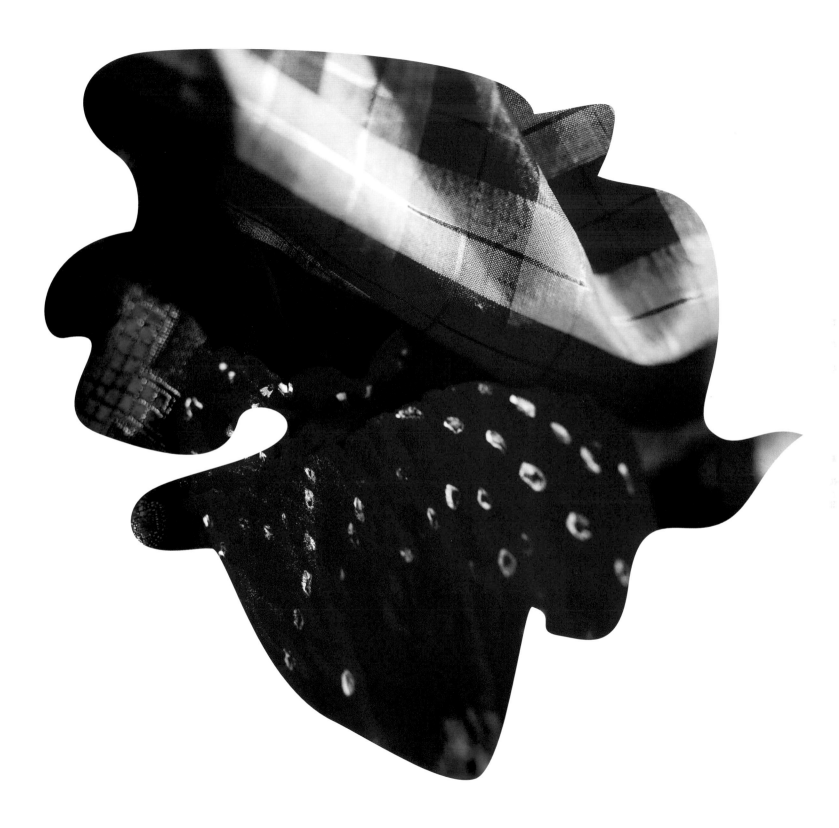

China

The Silk Route to China and the overland and sea routes to the East and Spice Islands were discovered in the pursuit of precious spice. The use of therapeutic plants was recorded in China long before the birth of Christ. In one of the oldest medical textbooks, written in 2000 B.C., the Chinese Emperor Kiwang-Ti described the medical properties of opium, rhubarb, and pomegranate. Between the Tang and Ming Dynasties (618–1644) the Chinese advanced culturally and technologically and played a hand in the development of the industrialized world. Papermaking, alcohol, printing, and porcelain all were featured in daily life. In China there was little distinction between drugs, spices, incense, and perfume. Substances that nurture the body and spirit were treated as one. Temples, houses, shops, and places of commerce were all scented sweetly with balms and essences. The wood camphor was used as a gastric stimulant and calmative in a herbal tea form. It was added to wine and used in cooking. The rosaries of Buddhist monks and nuns were carved out of the fine-grained wood, which became more lustrous with wear. Sutra chests were fashioned out of camphor because it deterred insects and protected fragile scrolls and books. The name "camphors," which often refers to solid oils, came from camphor, the most common solid.

Where would the world of flavor and fragrance be without citrus fruits? The tangerine, kumquat, Valencia, and Seville oranges came from China. The earliest references to citruses were in the *Nanfang ts'ao mu (Trees and Plants of the South)* written around A.D. 300 by Chi Han. Later, in the twelfth century, Chang Shih-na described placing orange flowers in a burner and heating them until "drops of liquid collect like sweat."

Peaches and apricots, both popular food and fragrance sources, also came from China and were collected and traded by Western merchants touring the Silk Route from Cathay.

The Chinese were interested in scenting the environment. Incense was burned around the clock, filling temples and homes with the heady fragrance. Incense symbolized the release from the mortal form to spirit and held enormous religious significance for the Chinese. However, recent research has discovered that they lack the glands responsible for body odor—the apocrine glands, which perhaps goes some way to explain the Chinese preoccupation with scenting the environment rather than the body. Aromatics to scent the skin were never all that important to Asians. Conversely, the apocrine glands under the armpits of Europeans form a largish bulb that emits powerful smells. As bathing was fashionable in the East, and not in the West, the need for the European to mask body odor was high on the list of social mores.

Porcelain made an important impact in the development of commercial essential oils. During the Sung Dynasty in the tenth century, the art of porcelain production was perfected, enabling Chinese alchemists to burn aromatics at high temperatures (porcelain is less reactive than glass). The Chinese also isolated the process of extracting ethyl alcohol from wine by cooling the condenser with cold water, thus advancing the distillation process. By the time Marco Polo arrived in China it was a busy urban civilization, with wondrous riches and advanced sciences. According to Edwin T. Morris, Marco Polo described Hangchou as "the greatest city in the world, where so many pleasures may be found that one fancies himself to be in Paradise." As developing trade routes and colonization contributed to the growth of Western culture, the mysteries of the East unfolded before the eyes, noses, and palates of the occidental world.

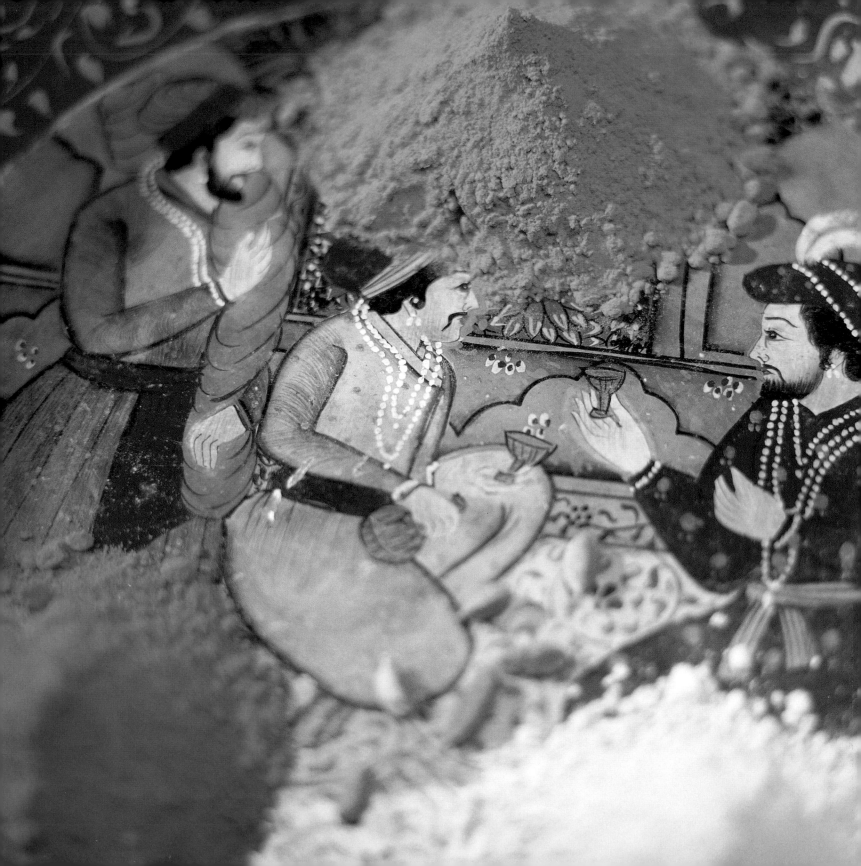

Europe

When the Roman empire fell in the fifth century A.D., little was left of the wisdom of the Greco-Roman culture. It wasn't until the returning crusaders and merchants learned of the healing and sensual arts of the East that the skills of distillation were brought back to Europe. The lust for land, money, spice, colonies, and trade opened the unenlightened minds of pre-Renaissance Europeans. However, the healing arts and sciences were left largely in the hands of monks cloistered away in monasteries during the Middle Ages.

In the tenth century, a university at Salerno emerged as a center of learning and botanical medicine. Constantius Africanus, an Arab from Baghdad, lectured in pharmacy, herbalism, and medicine. It was at this university that many experiments were performed to extract alcohol from wine. It was known as the "quintessence," the fifth essence that complemented water, air, fire, and earth. The key was a new and improved cooling device, borrowed from Arabic tradition, called the "Moors Head" cooling cap. Cardinal Vitalis de Furno declared the new essence to be a panacea for all ills and every university and pharmaceutical school began distilling the cure.

By the late Middle Ages apothecary guilds had been established in northern Europe. The essential oils and spices imported from the East enhanced the quality of life and improved the average European's chance of survival. The great plagues that swept through Europe ignited a surge of interest in alcohol and herbs as people discovered that alcohol was not tainted by disease and that perfumers, alchemists, and herbalists somehow escaped the scourge of the plagues.

By the fourteenth century plantations of lavender, rose, and sage were established in France, and by 1370 the first modern perfumes appeared. One early perfume, a basic combination of rosemary, lavender, and alcohol, known as "Hungary Water" after the Queen of Hungary, became famous. According to legend, this scent brought eternal youth and was said to have preserved the Queen's great beauty. The myth was fueled by a proposal from the King of Poland to the Queen when she was seventy-two years of age.

The illustrious Italian Medici family, who acquired much of their wealth through trade, made a fair living out of spice and aromatics. The royal family went to Provence every winter and a domestic industry for the production of floral fragrances began at Grasse, where the climate enabled roses, jasmine, violets, and acacia to flourish. Catherine de Medici, a famous sensualist, was always attended by her perfumer/chemist Signor Torabelli, who prepared creams and ointments to maintain her fair skin and the odd poisoned glove to dispose of her enemies. The Italians surpassed all Europeans in the manufacture and production of aromatics.

Florentine perfumes were used for everything from

eliminating body odor and firming flaccid breasts to restoring virginity. Perfumes were used to scent the breath and hair and were valuable skin tonics.

The antibacterial, antiviral properties brought relief to cancerous sores, rotting teeth, souring gums, and foul-smelling private parts.

It was not until the sixteenth century that the "Italianization" (the manners, arts, and sciences of Florence) pervaded French culture. Henri IV (1553–1610) resisted the new Italian ways, which he considered foppish; however, his friends said that "he stank like a carrion." Bathing was generally considered bad for the health. Fear of colds and fever, the cool climates of France, England, and Germany, and the prevalence of syphilis made people scorn bathing—still a public practice.

However, a movement emerged that considered hygiene and bodily adornment de rigueur. Louis XIV (1638–1715) was said to be so sensitive to smells that he had his perfumer concoct a special scent each day.

France developed as the perfume capital of Europe with Grasse and Montpellier supplying herbs all over Europe. Fields overflowing with medicinal herbs and flowers like carnations, violets, rose, lavender, jasmine, and tuberose became the stock-in-trade of the day. Wigs and handkerchiefs, nosegays (posies) and clothes were all scented with perfumes. In England Queen Elizabeth I was proud of her scented Spanish gloves and boasted of her stillroom, where fragrant waters were made for the courtiers. Shakespeare often alluded to the rose and mentions violets, marjoram, mint, lavender, and musk. He also spoke of the "casting bottle" used in Elizabethan times to scent a room.

The sixteenth century was the heyday of herbal medicine. Many of the essential oils used today were isolated by this time. This was the golden age of the English herbalist Nicholas Culpeper, who used plant essences to heal. He published several significant books on herbs and essences as well as a beauty manual called *Arts Master-Piece* (1660). The treatise is full of recipes, many of which employ resins, herbs, oils, and waters.

The Rococo period was a time of great excess, and perfume slowly moved away from its spiritual and medicinal origins and began its foray into the world of luxury and grandeur. In France, la Marquise de Pompadour, the Comtesse du Barry, and Marie Antoinette encouraged every facet of the decorative arts and their generous patronage profited perfumers from Grasse to Paris. Seventy firms were recognized as the creators of purely luxury goods—the *gantiers-parfumeurs*. The most famous scent of the fine kid gloves of the day was

"The olfactory sense has always been one of the most important tools of the chemist."
—Science historian Joseph Needham

neroli, named after the Duchess of Nerola. Scented gloves were one of the most coveted fragranced products of the time and it is said that when Queen Anne of Austria died she left no less than 340 pairs.

By 1789 the gap between the rich and poor had widened and a bridge could not be built to save France's customs of excess. The revolutionaries wanted nothing of perfume or luxury, wigs, elaborate dresses, or any of the accessories of nobility. Not a bad move considering many of the rich adornments of the day were disease carriers. It was not uncommon for rats, insects, and lice to live in the wigs, wardrobes, and clothes of the European illuminati.

It was not until Napoleon Bonaparte came to power in 1804 that many of the fine arts were revived in France and then encouraged in other parts of Europe. The new empire was characterized by a minirenaissance in the arts and sciences. In 1818 J. J. Houton de la Billardiere discovered the chemical patterns that underlie fragrant oils. His work was figured on that of J. B. Dumas (1800–1884), who investigated the makeup of many essential oils. In 1835, when H. E. Robiquet conducted the first successful experiments in the extraction of the essential oils of flowers that could not withstand distillation, solvent extraction was discovered.

Inspired by the remarkable advances in Napoleonic France, Germany became a center for the chemical sciences. In 1818 Romershausen performed the first distillation under a vacuum—a practice still used today in the manufacture of perfume and pharmaceuticals. Other German chemists pioneered the creation of synthetic fragrances.

By the nineteenth century scientific procedures and technology for procuring and testing botanical essences had become more refined. In 1882 William Whitla had published his materia medica, in which he discussed the known constituents and properties of twenty-five different essences. French researchers discovered that the tuberculosis bacillus could be deactivated by clove essence and that essence of thyme could help vanquish the typhus bacteria. But as the science of chemistry became more sophisticated, herbs were often abandoned in favor of more fashionable, synthetic drugs that acted quickly and powerfully. Apothecaries began to eliminate essences from their inventories, keeping only those useful as flavors and calmatives. Essential oils were relegated to the realm of perfumery, which is where they have principally remained. The age of miracle drugs separated botanical healing and the esoteric healing arts from their medicinal origins. Aromatherapy, the science of healing with essential oils, was not revived until the early twentieth century by René-Maurice Gattefossé.

"Victorian textile manufacturers discovered that their paisley designs would not sell unless they also had the patchouli fragrance of the Indian originals."
—Edwin T. Morris, *Fragrance: The Story of Perfume from Cleopatra to Chanel*

Modern aromatherapy

Gattefossé is often referred to as the father of modern aromatherapy, but there have been many others who have since contributed to the science and art of aromatherapy. Before WWII in Paris, the birthplace of modern aromatherapy, a medical doctor, Jean Valnet, revived Gattefossé's work. Charmed by the simple, natural cures, he devoted most of his time to experimenting with essential oils and recording the results. Valnet's work brought credibility and authority to the practice, and he published numerous books and articles that specifically addressed French medical traditions. His success spread far and wide as he treated many complex conditions with essential oils and other natural medicines. He employed classical methodology, and, due to his discipline and devotion, many medical aromatherapists followed in his footsteps. In France today many medical practitioners prescribe essential oils in place of drugs.

Earlier this century, Marguerite Maury, a charismatic Austrian biochemist and two-time winner of the Prix International d'Esthétique et Cosmétologie (an international prize awarded for exceptional scientific contributions to cosmetic research), developed a method of applying essential oils in massage. Madame Maury pioneered a technique whereby the oils were used to treat the body in a synergy of touch and smell—stimulating internal organs and improving the condition of the skin. Micheline Arcier is another figure who emerges as a key player in the establishment of modern aromatherapy. She studied under Madame Maury and Dr. Valnet and theorized that aromatherapy could be a complete holistic health system. The Micheline Arcier clinics, which implement her methods, are now famous all over the United Kingdom.

Essential oils and the flowering plants, herbs, and trees from which they are derived were universal medical tools for many centuries. It was not until synthetically manufactured substances were widely available that herbal medicine was put aside: Humanity believed it could not only tame the natural world but improve on it.

Aromatherapy is the art of treating the body with substances harvested from nature's rich store. It is an age-old practice that embraces the concepts of holistic healing, treatments that consider the mind, body, spirit, and emotions when making a diagnosis.

We can
no longer
separate ourselves
from nature, nor can
we ignore our impact
on the world around us.
By treating the body,
mind, and spirit
with nature's own
medicines, we bring
harmony and
balance to
life.

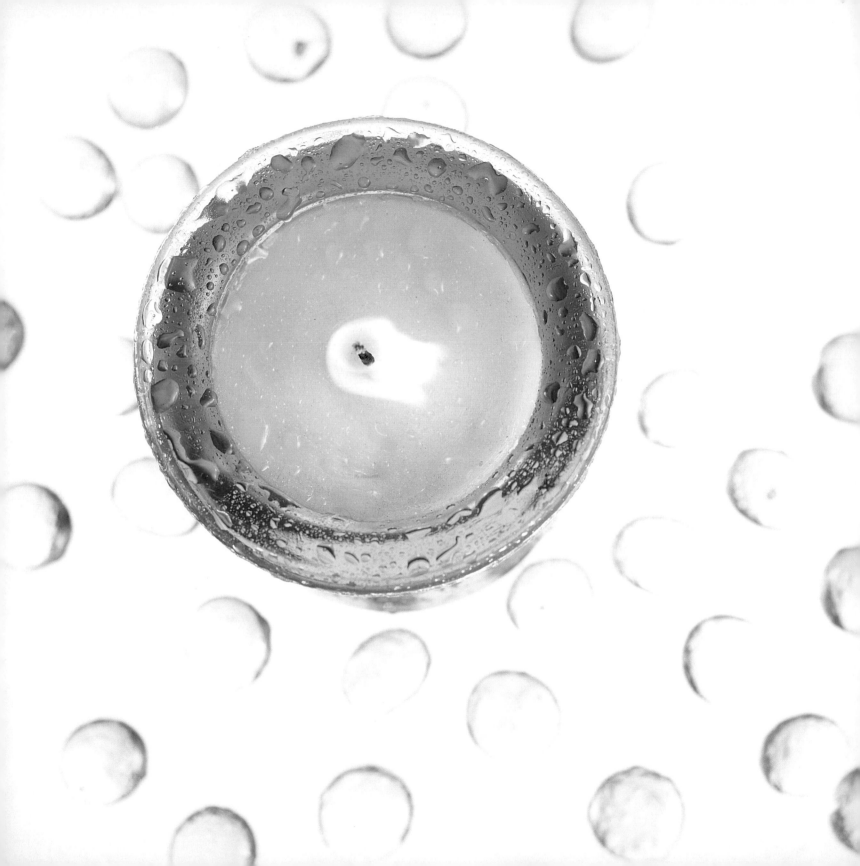

natural mechanics

How aromatherapy works on your mind, body, and spirit

When Marguerite Maury, a brilliant French biochemist and body-worker, developed her unique form of applying essential oils with massage in France in the early 1920s, a doorway to sensual healing opened to the world. A new branch of aromatherapy—applying the oils in a synergy of touch and smell—meant that aromatherapy became accessible to everyone. No longer the exclusive domain of herbalists, alchemists, and doctors, essential oils could now be used by all people wishing to treat themselves.

Today, the term "aromatherapist" generally applies to someone trained in the use of essential oils. Qualifications vary. Some are trained in the biochemistry of the oils and their actions on the human body, some specialize in using aromatherapy to treat psychological and emotional conditions, while others understand their cosmetic properties and apply essential oils in beauty treatments. In France, many doctors and naturopaths prescribe essential oils for internal use, but these practitioners have had very specific training.

Modern aromatherapy provides us with a contemporary version of an ancient healing science. Aromatherapy is based on the idea that you can maintain health by boosting the body's own defense mechanisms via touch and smell. Aromatherapy helps restore the harmony between the body, mind, and outside world—a harmony that is continually disrupted by pollution, stress, busy schedules, and all the rigors of modern existence. Aromatherapy can have a positive impact on the way you look, think, and feel, revealing pathways to a fuller, richer life.

Penetration

Essential oils are extracted from plants. They are natural chemical substances that evaporate quickly when exposed to the air—which is why we can smell them. They are called essential oils after the Latin word *essentia*, meaning "essence," a liquid that easily becomes gaseous. Because they vaporize quickly, the essential oils are also known as volatile or spirit oils, from the Latin *volare*, "to fly"—the human nose knows they are present in the air even when they are no longer visible as a liquid. These complex organic chemicals are soluble in vegetable oil and alcohol. Essential oils enter the body via the skin and nose. When the tiny molecules are inhaled or massaged into the skin, they penetrate the bloodstream and act on the organs within the body.

Our sense of smell

Of all the body's faculties, the sense of smell is surely the least appreciated. Helen Keller, whose own nose was so sensitive she could smell approaching rain, believed "smell was the fallen angel of the senses." Her blindness from the age of nineteen months led her sense of smell to develop far greater sensitivity than that of sighted people. Even an average nose can detect the scent of a few stray molecules hovering in the atmosphere—a highly sophisticated chemical accomplishment. Fragrance and food are intimately linked. In fact, food is reduced to blandness and texture only without the nose, as the tongue can only distinguish salty, bitter, sweet, and sour—without smell it's impossible to tell the difference between the crunch of apples and onions. Our sense of smell is sometimes known as the mute sense. Although incredibly precise, it's almost impossible to describe a smell to someone who hasn't smelled it. The smell of new shoes, for example, or the smell of moldy oranges, the scent of the sea or the smell of your lover are impossible to describe. We smell with every breath. As we breathe in we invite the outside world into our inner universe; when we exhale we give a minute amount of ourselves back to the environment in the form of gas. One whiff of perfume can bring back a flood of memories so vivid it can bring tears to the eyes or joy to the heart because a direct physical route exists between memory and smell, adroitly transporting us through time and distance. But, despite their impressive powers, most urban noses have been in a state of olfactory decline for centuries. Researchers speculate that because humans no longer need to smell to survive, the nose has been superseded by other senses, whereas our distant ancestors were designed as virtual smelling machines and relied on smell to choose partners and identify foods and prospective enemies. Smell is still a vital part of reproduction for many mammals including mice and chimpanzees. Male odors actually "invite" ovulation, and the scent of the female helps prepare the male for copulation. In laboratory experiments scientists have interfered with the nasal nerves, which takes away the animal's sexual urge. Without smell there is no offspring and no perpetuation of the species. A combination of underuse, pollution, mucus-producing diets, and cigarette smoke has caused a considerable degeneration in our sense of smell. Today, however, we are on the brink of an olfactory renaissance. For the first time in history scientists are seriously researching and documenting the power of smell and its long-baffling fundamental chemistry. In universities and research institutions, scientists are discovering the vital connection between smell and health, nutrition, psychology, and the olfactory holy grail—human pheromones.

The physiology of smell

At birth we experience life as breath; it's our first taste of the world. At death we sigh out the last moment of life. During the average life span a person breathes about 23,040 times. It takes about five seconds to breathe—two seconds to inhale and three to exhale. All the time we are breathing, we are smelling. The olfactory epithelium, the small patch at the top of the nasal cavity, contains about five million receptor cells that can recognize about 10,000 different smells. Much information processing is done by the olfactory bulb in the roof of the nasal cavity, and from there the results are fired directly to the brain's limbic system. The limbic system is the seat of memory and emotion and is designed to interpret pleasant and unpleasant stimuli. It is here that the brain translates memory into chemical messages. In the limbic system smell, emotion, and memory are intimately linked. When the olfactory bulb detects a scent—a food, a lover, a flower—it signals the brain and sends a message straight into the limbic system, crossing time and space barriers. The effect is so immediate we barely have time to translate the data into memory pictures and feelings. As Edwin T. Morris points out in *Fragrance*, "there's almost no short-term memory with odors." Morris also notes that smells can be used to stimulate learning and retention. "When children were given olfactory information along with a word list, the list was recalled much more easily and better retained in memory than when given without olfactory cues." Smells are memory catalysts. The Russian novelist Vladimir Nabokov remarked, "Nothing revives the past so completely as smell." Smell, along with taste, is a chemical response. It enjoys a molecular relationship with other parts of the body, which is the reason why an unpleasant smell can instantly make you nauseated, sending a wave of chemical messages to the stomach, or why a yummy smell can make you hungry, producing a complex chain of chemical reactions that stimulate gastric juices and make the mouth water. Musk, which is chemically similar to human testosterone, can be detected in minuscule portions and can produce an extraordinary hormonal change in the woman who smells it. Smells from one individual can also shift hormone levels in another. Scientists have discovered that women who live together find their menstrual cycles become synchronized over time, a feat most likely accomplished by smell. It may also be that when we say that an atmosphere is "heavy," that we are actually smelling fear or depression. We all have a genetically encoded "odor print" that is as individual as our fingerprints. Only identical twins smell alike. Smells identify us, which is one of the reasons why our sense of smell remains very important to our well-being. An infant makes an olfactory bond with its mother within three days of birth. The sexual and emotional bonding between mates is associated with the hormonal processes of the limbic center in the brain—every lover knows the ecstasy of their beloved's scent. And it takes only 0.5 seconds for humans to respond to a smell, compared with 0.9 seconds to react to pain. Smell still alerts us to spoiled food or poison gas: It is one of our most powerful protective mechanisms.

Researchers have discovered that anosmia, or smell blindness, which affects approximately one in a million people, is a sometimes dangerous and very debilitating condition. Anosmics often lose their appetite for life, becoming depressed, impotent, and introverted.

Lock and key

Around 60 B.C. the Roman poet Lucretius wrote a tome on the world as he saw it called *The Nature of Things*. He proposed that the reactions between things in the universe worked with a sort of lock and key mechanism. This was expanded in 1949 by J. E. Amoore's "stereochemical theory," which maps the connections between geometric shapes of molecules and the odor sensations they produce. According to the theory, if a molecule of the right shape fits into a neuron niche, it will trigger a nerve impulse in the brain. For example, researchers speculate that minty odors have wedge-shaped molecules that fit into V-shaped sites and musky odors have disc-shaped molecules that fit into elliptical, bowl-like sites on the neuron. Amoore's work remains theory but he was not too far off the mark. The most popular theory today is that different proteins will bind only with the molecules of certain odors, setting off a chain reaction of chemical changes that the brain registers as a particular smell. Tiny hairs protrude from the nerve cells at the back of the fibers on the nasal epithelium that are rich in the receptor proteins needed to register odor. Using the same lock and key explanation, these receptors have a specific shape that match the shape of particular smells.

When the peppermint-shaped protein receptors are fully occupied, for example, there is nothing in the nose for the peppermint molecules to fit into and we cannot smell them, however many are pumped into the nostrils. This is why we often lose the ability to smell fragrance on ourselves soon after we apply it. After a while, scent molecules are probably metabolized by the body. We can smell them again once the key is out of the lock—or once the receptors are no longer occupied. This theory may also explain olfactory blind spots: why some people can't smell garlic and some people can't smell musk. The receptor sites for those particular smells may not be present on the nerve cells of the nasal fibers. The lock and key as a metaphor for aromatherapy is very potent.

Essential oils have an extraordinary effect on physiology. Inhaling natural substances is an exquisite, complex, profound, seductive, mysterious, and primitive experience. Perhaps botanical smells excite us because they spring from nature herself. Smells of flowers and plants seem to unlock a part of the human brain that is wild—close to the earth, its seasons, its rhythms, and its optimistic, uncontained fecundity and robust energy.

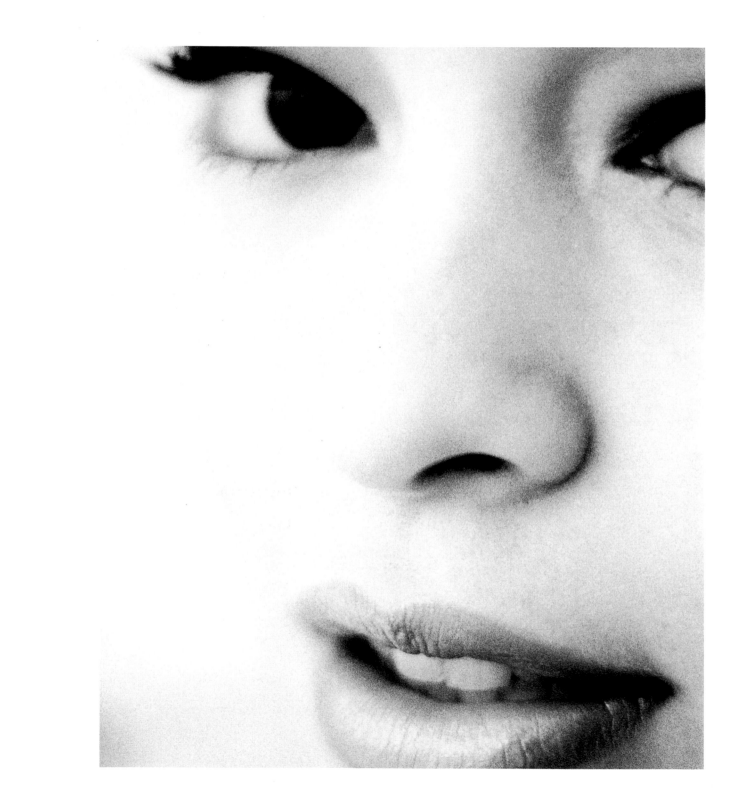

Inhalation

One of the great joys of aromatherapy is that the pleasure is experienced by anyone who inhales the aromas. Whether oils are burned and infused into the atmosphere, stroked in with healing massage, or simply wafted under the nose, a significant concentration of odor molecules reaches the inner sanctum of the nose.

Currents of air carry aromatic substances to the olfactory epithelium in the brain and although the area for absorption is some 4,000 times smaller than that of the skin, the registration

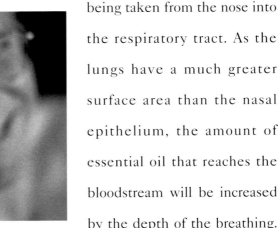

of smells is high. Substances absorbed via the nasal mucosa have direct access to the central nervous system, and essential oils absorbed through the lining of the nose certainly reach the brain. Inhaled molecules pass down the trachea into the bronchi, and from there into finer bronchioles, completing their journey at the microscopic, saclike alveoli of the lungs, where gaseous exchange with the blood takes place. These alveoli are extremely efficient at transporting small molecules, like essential oil constituents, into the blood, which carries them to other parts of the body. Whether essential oils are sniffed directly from the bottle, breathed in through the air, or simply inhaled during massage, aromatherapy treatments result in molecules being taken from the nose into the respiratory tract. As the lungs have a much greater surface area than the nasal epithelium, the amount of essential oil that reaches the bloodstream will be increased by the depth of the breathing.

Most aromatherapists believe greater absorption into the bloodstream enhances the effects of the oil.

Anecdotal reports of the mood-altering effects of inhaling scent imply that when essential oils penetrate the bloodstream and reach the limbic center of the brain, they alter the chemistry of the body.

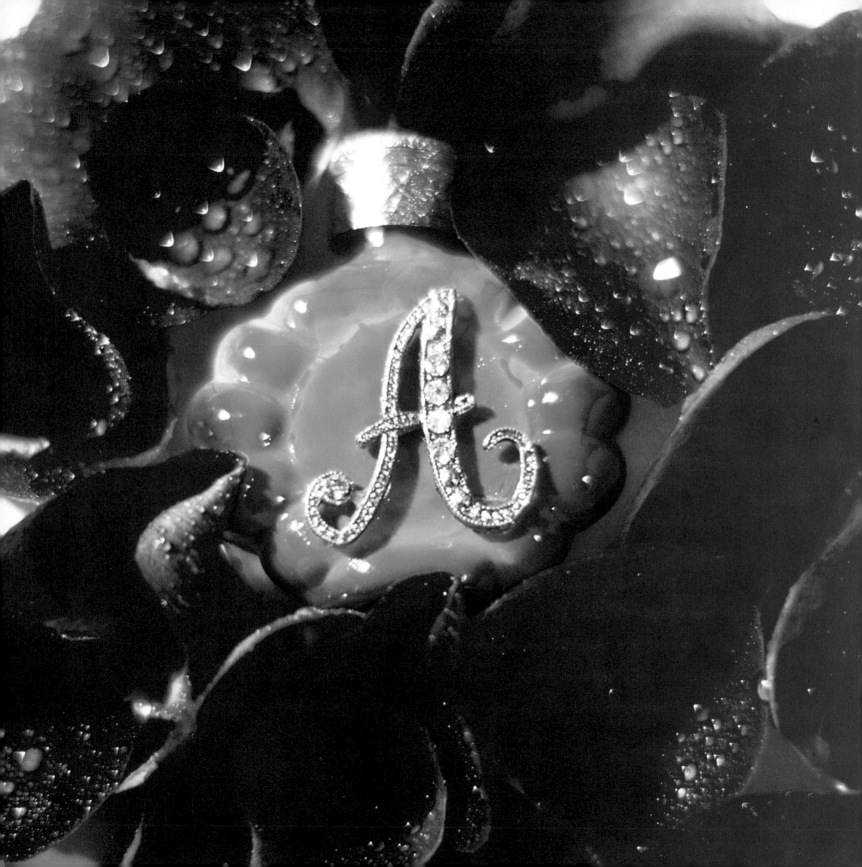

Scientists at the Memorial Sloan-Kettering Cancer Center in New York have discovered the vanillalike smell of heliotropin can help reduce patient anxiety when undergoing stressful examinations like magnetic resonance imaging (MRI).

Japanese researchers have discovered that lemon essence helps cut rates of error by computer operators by up to 50 percent.

The Japanese firm Shimizu deploys a woody scent to soften the mood in the banquet room of its headquarters.

Touch

A baby cradled in its mother's arms already knows the pleasure of touch. The sensations of comfort and security envelop the child as it is held close, absorbing the warmth, feeling its mother's breath and heartbeat. For a fetus in the mother's womb, touch is the first sense to develop and it is through this crucial ability to "feel" that the newborn child learns about pleasure and pain.

Most modern humans touch and are touched infrequently in day-to-day life. We receive more sensations through our eyes and ears than through our skin. We touch fabric, we touch nature, we touch buttons and keyboards, and we reserve intimate touches for the bedroom. Doctors touch patients as little as possible. Traditionally, Western healing hands have had more contact with prescription pads than aching bodies, yet recent research shows that even minimal physical contact between patient and physician before surgery can dramatically affect recovery. Patients whose hands are held by their doctors for as little as thirty seconds before an operation often leave intensive care units sooner than noncontact patients.

People who aren't touched enough suffer from emotional deprivation. Geriatric studies show that senility in the elderly is often a response to sensual starvation and can be reversed when they are stroked and caressed. Orphaned baby monkeys have been known to self-mutilate when deprived of touch, and on a human level, infants deprived of touch will become emotionally retarded, psychologically starved, and physically wasted. When given only a minimum of care—food, clean clothing, and nothing more—the result is an underdeveloped individual, susceptible to immune deficiency and with poor chances of survival. Ezra Pound once said D. H. Lawrence's use of the word "touch" isn't epidermal, but encompasses the profound penetration into the core of someone's being. Touch, like smell, bypasses the logical mind and plumbs the depths of the soul. Lovers know the importance of touch, as do healers. We never grow out of the need to be touched, but as we grow up in our society it's harder to get. In dramatic contrast to the stiff handshake of Westerners, Eskimos and Maoris greet strangers by pressing or rubbing noses. And in Africa and India villagers happily gather around a stranger for an exploratory touch.

Touch has taboos. A kiss, a caress, a slap, a brush can all mean different things at different times. There's no such thing as an inappropriate smell, but inappropriate touch is something society abhors. A friend's lover may kiss you on the cheek but when that kiss is on the lips it means something else. Perhaps in an attempt to control inappropriate touch, Western society has shunned it, hidden it beneath clothes and behind closed doors. Touch has been relegated to the boudoir or at least the confines of the family. Even then, fathers tend to stop kissing their sons at an early age and mothers also tend to touch their children less as they reach adolescence. Touch is, however, a part of being human, and an essential part of health and well-being. Massage is a terrific way to touch people. A simple head or foot massage can remove all the strains of the day. Giving a hand massage to a colleague can change a work relationship entirely. Aromatherapy massage is a gift worth giving—hands are the messengers of love, care, and compassion.

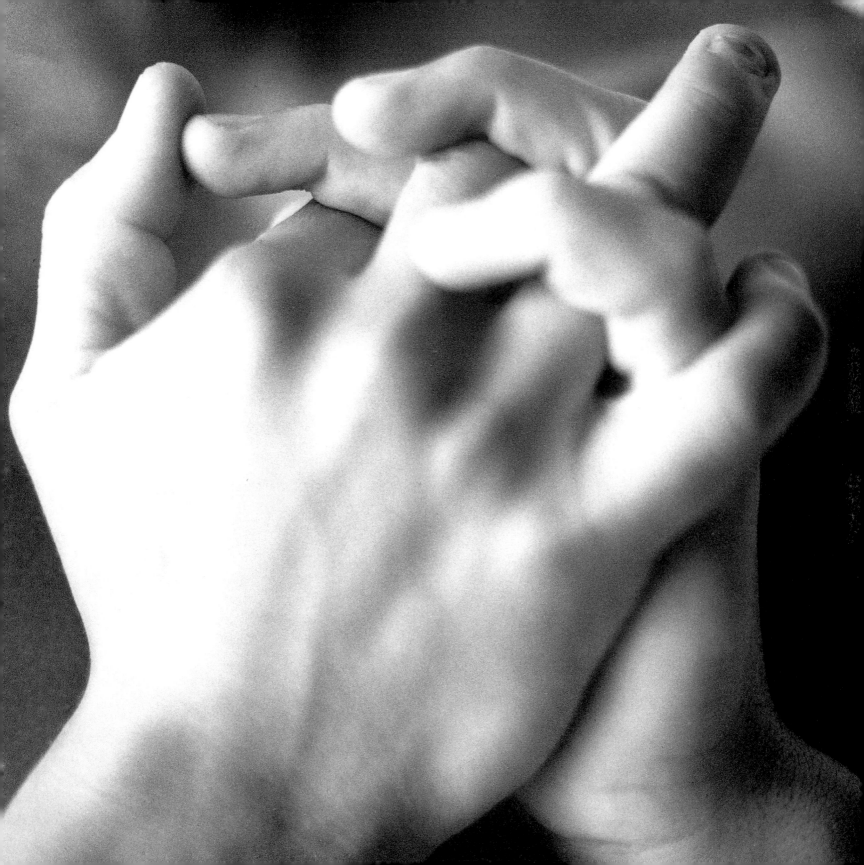

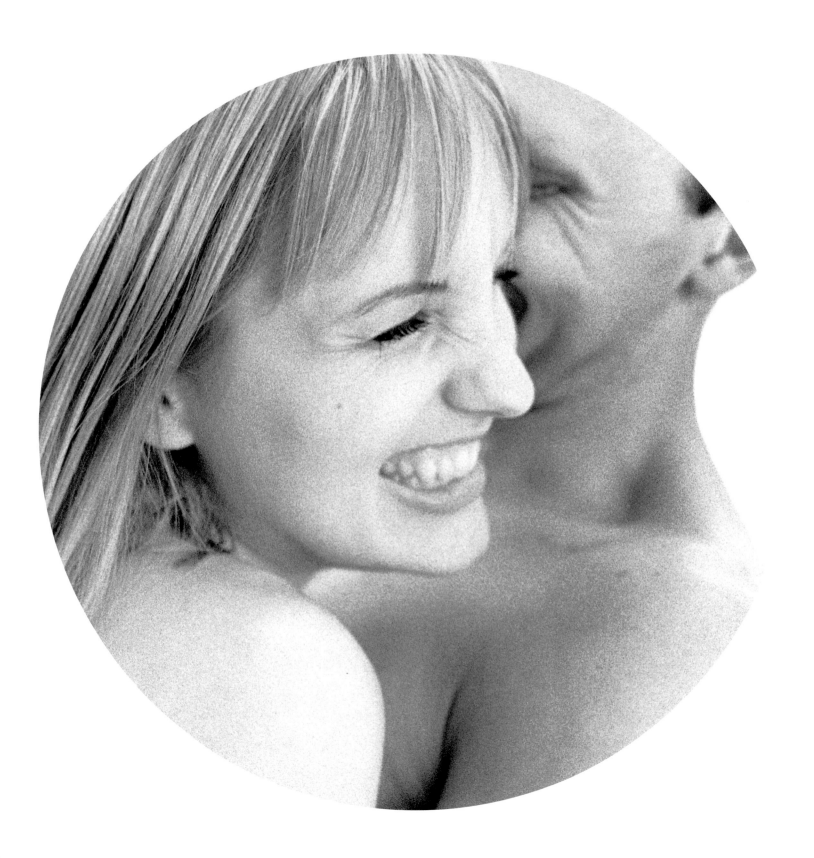

The physiology of touch

The skin is made for touch. Nature intended the skin to produce sensation. The feeling of touch is transmitted to the brain through an elaborate network of touch receptors and nerve endings on and under the skin in the form of electrical charges. This highly charged network makes our sense of touch extremely sensitive. Some touch receptors will react in less than a tenth of a second. The fingertips, soles of the feet, lips, tongue, palms, and the sexual zones, such as the nipples, clitoris, and penis, have highly sensitive receptors programmed to register pleasure and pain in a millisecond. Hairy parts of the skin are supersensitive because each hair is rooted in a follicle that is surrounded by a nerve—the downy fuzz on a woman's cheek is far more sensitive than the guard hairs or coarse hairs on the arms and legs. Because the skin is so sensitive to touch it can convey messages to the rest of the body, which is why massage is able to improve gland, circulation, organ, and nerve function while relaxing muscles and sending healing bliss-inducing chemicals to the brain. Touch receptors become conditioned with repetition. The hardness and chill of a cold wristwatch is felt by our skin, but in time we forget we are wearing it. When a change occurs, like taking the watch off, receptors shoot new messages to the brain to alert it to the change in conditions. If that on/off switch didn't work the nervous system would become overloaded with the sensations of touch. We'd never be able to wear a wool sweater or be able to cope with water beating down in a shower. Touch is pleasurable when the movements change from a tickle to a caress or a pinch to a stroke. No other sense can arouse you like touch. In her book, *A Natural History of the Senses*, Diane Ackerman quotes American neurologist Saul Schanberg, who said, "If touch didn't feel good, there'd be no species, parenthood, or survival. A mother wouldn't touch her baby in the right way unless she felt pleasure doing it. If we didn't like the feel of touching and patting one another, we wouldn't have had sex. Those animals who did more touching instinctively produced offspring which survived, and their genes were passed on and the tendency to touch became even stronger. We forget that touch is not only basic to our species, but the key to it."

Aromatherapy comes into its own in the arena of touch. When essential oils are stroked, caressed, and gently massaged into the skin, the nervous system is stimulated, the internal organs are treated, the senses are aroused, the emotions are soothed, and the spirit soars.

Aromatherapy massage is a gift worth giving—hands are the messengers of love, care, and compassion. "Touch fills our memory with a detailed key as to how we are shaped. A mirror would mean nothing without touch. We are forever taking the measure of ourselves in unconscious ways—idly running one hand along a forearm, seeing if our thumb and forefinger can bracelet our wrist or if we can touch our tongue to our nose or bend our thumb all the way back . . . nervously twisting a strand of hair. But, above all, touch teaches us that life has depth and contour; it makes our sense of the world and ourself three dimensional. Without that intricate feel for life there would be no artists, whose cunning is to make sensory and emotional maps, and no surgeons, who dive through the body with their fingertips." —Diane Ackerman, *A Natural History of the Senses*

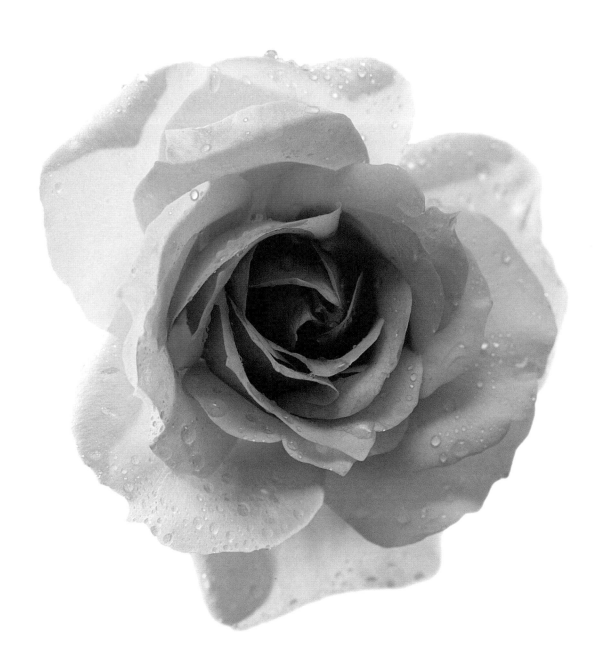

The skin

The skin is the largest organ of the body. This attractive and practical wrapping covers the entire body surface and contains blood vessels, thousands of nerve endings, hundreds of sweat glands, and millions of cells. The primary function of the skin is to protect. It functions as a living, breathing suit of armor that keeps all our vital organs safely inside and environmental enemies outside. This complex organ eliminates waste, manufactures vitamins, and through thousands of sensory nerve endings, warns us of danger and informs us of pleasure. The skin is also responsible for growing hairs and regulating the body's temperature. It absorbs substances like a sponge into its deeper layers, which can be both harmful and beneficial.

Essential oils penetrate the skin through a process known as diffusion. In contrast to sweating, which is an active, energy-demanding process, the passage of essential oil molecules inward through the skin occurs quite passively—the skin cells don't actually pump the substances down into the deeper layers of the skin, they sink in naturally. How much is diffused depends on the surface area to which the substance is applied. Basically, the more skin you cover with essential oils, the greater the dose. Some oils will effectively treat conditions in very small amounts. This is important when it comes to using very strong oils in massage—it's possible to overdose on some oils.

Molecules of essential oils pass through the skin's epidermis and are carried away by the capillary blood circulating in the dermis below. Studies have found that heat and water can enhance the permeability of essential oils. For example, oil of wintergreen is absorbed much more quickly when the skin is prepared with water before application, and the warm hands of an aromatherapist are said to speed the transfer of essential oils through the skin.

Where do they go?

Essential oils are dynamic, active, and highly sensitive substances that act quickly when applied to the body, diffusing through the skin and penetrating the walls of blood vessels and body tissues. Essential oils scatter and set up camp for a period of time in various regions of the body, then become metabolized and excreted. Although they do not remain in the body for more than three or four hours, they can trigger a healing process that can continue for days or weeks.

Essential oils dissolve readily into fat and

"Odiferous matter reached regions of the brain which are not under conscious control; its

pass easily into the central nervous system and the liver. The brain is very rich in fats; therefore fat-soluble molecules like essential oils will be taken up easily by the brain and remain there for some time. Many essential oil molecules gain rapid entry to the central nervous system via the blood-brain barrier. This barrier acts as a screen, protecting the brain from many toxic chemicals. Recent studies have shown that various constituents of essential oils penetrate the blood-brain barrier and have fairly significant mood-altering effects. For example, several of the constituents of nutmeg are potentially convertible to chemicals similar to hallucinogens. Melissa and lavender have been found to have marked sedative effects. Once essential oils are absorbed into the body a whole range of chemical transformations takes place.

The body loves the protective and preventive properties of the oils and marshals their support to help prevent attack from bacteria, viruses, fungi, parasites, allergens, and toxins. For example, tea tree oil is a very effective and nonharmful antimicrobial essential oil. It helps destroy *Candida albicans*, the fungus that causes thrush, and can kill *Trichomonas vaginalis*, a tiny creature often responsible for vaginal infections, without hurting or unbalancing the body. Because essential oil molecules are small and organic, researchers assume that essential oils and drugs are treated by the body in a similar way—but without many of the damaging side effects of synthetically made drugs. In its brilliant and efficient way, the body knows how to make the most of the vital properties of essential oils to bring itself into balance and well-being.

Feeling

It is quite easy to explain the chemical effects of essential oils on the body and brain, but it is much harder to dissect and quantify the effects of essential oils on the emotional and spiritual aspects of life. For the last few hundred years Western society has looked to medicine and science to cure everything from cancer to depression. We believed doctors had all the answers and attributed them with godlike powers to heal. But in recent years, many people have become disillusioned with modern medicine and have turned to alternative therapies, such as aromatherapy, to treat physiological and emotional complaints. While aromatherapy is a science of biochemistry, it is also an "esoteric" practice, with some aromatherapists using essential oils to treat the mind and

perception affects our psychic life and transforms our predispositions." —Marguerite Maury

emotions first and foremost. We know that in basic, physical terms the constituents of essential oils can have an effect on the chemistry of the body, but we don't really know how or why the smell of ylang-ylang can set one person's spirits soaring and do nothing at all for another, or why lavender massaged lovingly into the feet of an old woman can lift long-term depression. There is something in the human soul that longs to be touched, to be pampered with sweet smelling oils, and that responds instantly, profoundly, to natural substances. Per-haps we can explain this phenomenon with calculations, science and biology, but there is something wonderful, magical, and spiritual in simply accept-ing that essential oils affect us on a level that cannot be easily explained by conventional scientific methods.

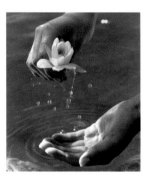

One cannot help thinking that the range and com-plexity of emotions experienced by humans is more than a little chemical exchange in the brain. Aromatherapy is a feel-good therapy immediately appreciated by anyone who has ever picked up a flower and sniffed its wondrous aroma.

In his book *Jitterbug Perfume*, Tom Robbins wrote: "Squeezed from the reproductive glands of plants and creatures, perfume is the smell of creation, a sign dramatically delivered to our senses of the Earth's regenerative powers—a message of hope and a message of pleasure." Essential oils are nature's perfumes and nature's medicines. The famous aromatherapist Robert Tisserand says "aromatherapy is a form of energy medicine." By energy medicine he means that the actions of essential oils work on a level deeper than that of the material body—a level you can't see or touch —only feel.

Aromatherapy has been used in religious rites, alchemical practices, magic, and healing since ancient times. Aromatherapists all over the world have seen and recorded the effects of essential oils on the mind, emotions, and body. Aromatics have been widely used in love potions and aphrodisiacs for centuries and have recently been shown to have powerful euphoric properties. Every lover knows that sex and depression simply don't mix and that feeling good brings on the sexual urge. Robert Tisserand reports that by treating impotent and frigid patients with jasmine, ylang-ylang, and clary sage he can whip up a sexual storm that breaks even the most persistent drought.

Conventional medicine is just catching on to the idea that you can't cure illness and disease by treating the body alone. The whole being must be taken into consideration. Doctors and therapists need to treat the mind and emotions as well as the

"The fragrance that came to each was like a memory of dewy mornings, of unshadowed sun, of which the fair world in spring is but a fleeting memory."

—J. R. R. Tolkien, *Lord of the Rings*

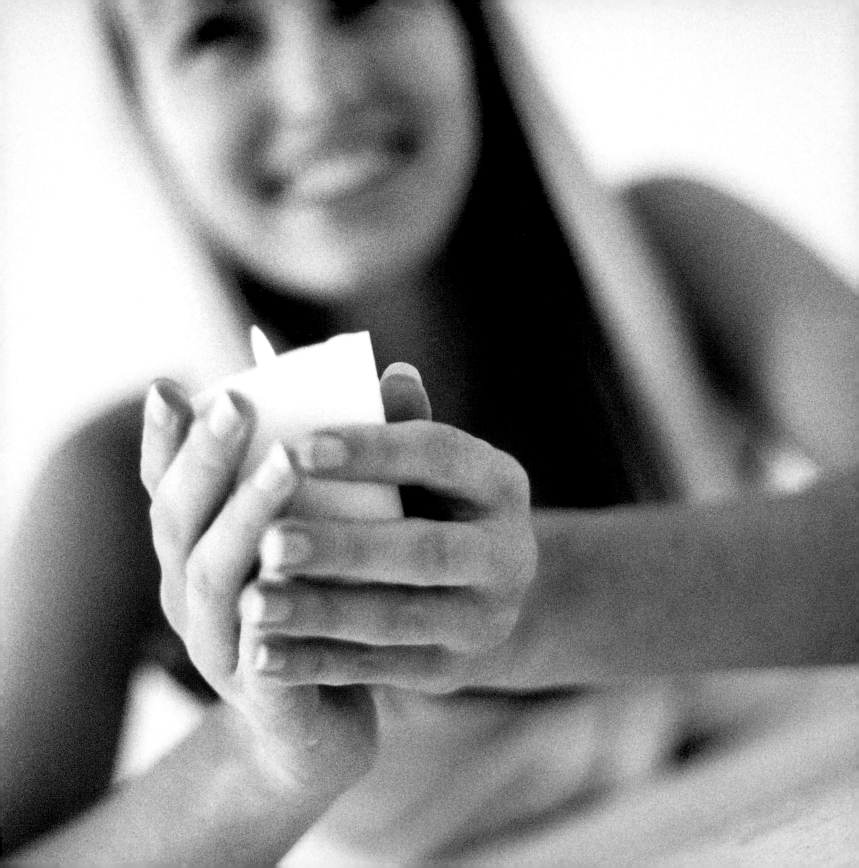

body if people are to be truly well and happy. Aromatherapy is a holistic therapy. It treats the feelings and spirit with the same respect as the physical body. When an aromatherapist prescribes lavender to sedate an anxious person who is afraid of losing his or her job, the therapist knows that on the physical level, lavender will treat the heart, boost the immune system, relieve any gastric or intestinal trouble, soothe irritable nerves, and ensure that the respiratory system is functioning normally. On the spiritual and emotional level, lavender will help elevate the spirits and give the person confidence and peace of mind. Essential oils work synergistically with the human body, treating the whole being—mind, body, and spirit.

Aromatherapy is also about relationships. It tends to the needs of the individual by offering simple, accessible solutions to some of the stresses of modern-day life. Treating yourself with essential oils opens a fragrant haven from the world where the mind, emotions, and body can unwind and relax. In doing so, aromatherapy allows you to go quietly within to treat and pamper yourself. Aromatherapy can also open the relationship between lovers and friends, as well as therapists and patients. In the same way that a friendly smile, a loving touch, or a compassionate word can heal many ills, the relationship between the healer and the client can be profound and life enhancing.

Aromatherapy pays homage to nature, celebrates the majesty of the human body, and respects the individual. No two people will have the same experiences, no two people will respond to the same smells, no two people have the same body chemistry. Aromatherapy is a very private joy that can be shared by two individuals for the betterment of both. Feelings may be fleeting and as changeable as the weather, but good feelings in high doses are the best medicine of all.

Aromatherapy is an incredibly broad healing discipline because it encompasses treatment through smell, touch, and feeling. Essential oils have an amazing affinity with the human body. Whether they are inhaled, massaged into the skin, worn as perfume or dabbed onto a wound, the tiny active molecules go to work, balancing and healing the body.

"Your
body is the river
of life that sustains you,
yet it does so humbly,
without asking for recognition. If
you sit and listen to it, you will find
that a powerful intelligence dwells
within you. It isn't an intelligence of
words, but compared to the millions
of years of wisdom woven into one
cell, the knowledge of words
doesn't seem so grand."
—Deepak Chopra, *Ageless
Body, Timeless Mind*

"Natural
therapies have become
known as 'listening therapies,'
where practitioners try to discover the
reason behind the body's cry for help, which
manifests itself in the form of headaches,
stomach upsets and breathing
problems." —Shirley
Price, *Aromatherapy
Workbook*

"It is evident that
natural odors are necessary
for our optimum spiritual well-being.
It is also clear that pleasant odors in
themselves are not as effective as essential
oils used in a therapeutic context. You can
bottle essential oils, but not aromatherapy."
—Robert Tisserand, *Aromatherapy
for Everyone*

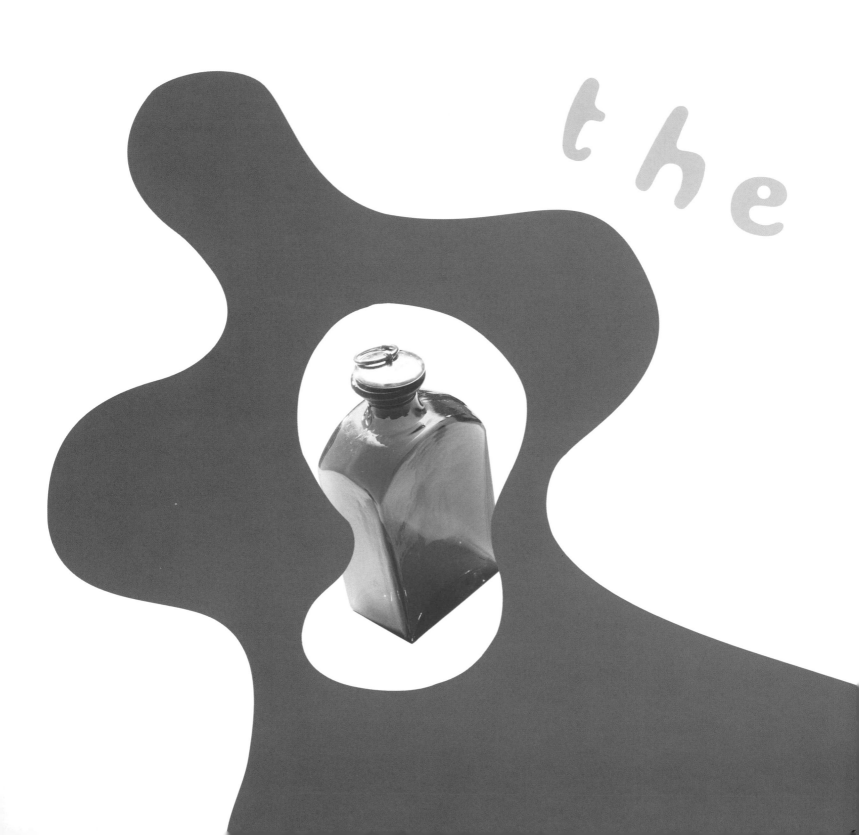

the

good oils

the lifeblood of aromatherapy—essential oils

Each essential oil has its own wondrous smell and healing magic. This comprehensive explanation of the most common oils reveals their history, individual characteristics, and use in treating minor ailments.

Extracting the essence

Pure essential oils are extracted from the bark, roots, berries, flowers, stalks, leaves, and resins of trees and plants. Early humans discovered the medicine in plants by eating them and applying them directly to wounds. As the knowledge of their healing benefits developed, flowers and plants were made into teas, poultices, tinctures, and ointments. Processes of distillation advanced and methods of extracting the magic became widely known and used. Although the basic principles for extracting essential oils from plants remain unchanged, even after hundreds of years, the methods and techniques employed today are amazingly proficient and economical.

Steam distillation

Steam distillation is the most common form of extracting essential oils. Plant materials are placed in a deep vat and steam is sent through the entire contents. Essential oils are contained in the glands, veins, sacs, and glandular hairs of aromatic plants. When the cell walls are ruptured by heat, tiny molecules evaporate and leave the plant. The molecules are carried in the steam along a pipe to cool and condense into liquid, and as they reach the end of the journey, they separate. Finally, the water is drawn off the oil and the result is a pure, natural essential oil.

Maceration

Maceration is an ancient method of extracting the "goodies" from plants and flowers. The Egyptians used this method to make pomades and cosmetics, macerating, or soaking, aromatic plants in animal fats and vegetable oils. Wooden frames with glass plates on top are laid out and covered with a mixture of animal fat and vegetable oil. Petals are spread evenly over the grease and replaced every few days until the fat is impregnated with scent. The fat is then washed with pure grain alcohol, which dissolves the essential oil compounds, leaving the fat behind. The essential oil and alcohol mixture is then vacuum distilled to remove the alcohol. What is left is known as the absolute. This method is generally employed when the aromatic components of the plant are sensitive to heat degradation or when the plant only provides a low yield of essential oil, like tuberose and jasmine. This method of extraction is rarely used today because it is labor-intensive and costly. Most floral absolutes are now produced using petrochemical solvents.

Enfleurage

Enfleurage is a process that involves soaking plants in warm oils until their precious essential oil is expressed into a carrier oil.

Expression

Expression is a method used exclusively to extract essential oils from citrus fruits. The vital citrus oils are located in sacs under the surface of the rind. When the peel is mechanically pressed, droplets of oil and juice are squeezed out and separated.

Solvent extraction

Solvent extraction generally refers to the extraction of aromatic compounds using hydrocarbon solvents. This method is usually employed for essences that have sensitive fragrances and low yields. Plant materials are placed in an extractor and washed with solvents. Since the boiling point of the solvents is lower than that of the essential oil, the solvent can be completely removed. This yields a concrete, a thick material that contains the plant oils, colors, and waxes. Grain alcohol is added to the concrete to remove the aromatic compounds, leaving the waxes and colors behind. Solvent extraction captures the true-to-life aroma of the plant or flower, but the solvents used can be toxic and dangerous. Some aromatherapists will not use essential oils extracted with solvents, because they believe the petrochemicals contaminate the pure substances, affecting both the aroma and the therapeutic benefits. It takes a fairly keen sense of smell to detect solvents in essential oils, but the best way to judge is by comparison. A slight petroleum smell may be detected in the background of a solvent-extracted scent.

Synthetics

During the latter part of the nineteenth century, the science of organic chemistry began to flourish, and scientists discovered that compounds that mimicked living organisms could be created in the laboratory. Synthetic smells were born. For the voracious flavors and fragrance industry, this was an enormous leap forward. It meant that it was possible to make something smell and taste like peppermint or gardenia without having to use the real ingredients.

Because we have become used to the idea that certain smells and tastes should always stay the same—such as your favorite fragrance, deodorant, or toothpaste—synthetic fragrances and flavors have been used extensively in the making of perfumes, food products, and toiletries. No two harvests are ever the same, so maintaining quality and scent is extremely difficult with natural substances, especially when you throw in environmental wild cards like drought, acid rain, and insect infestation. Synthetics can always be relied on to produce an identical smell or taste time after time.

In the case of musk, one of the most popular perfume bases, synthetic technology has saved a potentially endangered species. The *Moschus moschiferus* is a deer that lives in Central Asia. The male carries a small sac in the front of his abdomen that secretes a musky fluid similar to both a tomcat's spray and human testosterone. These secretions can be collected painlessly from the deer, but it is easier and cheaper to kill the animal and take the scent from the sac. There is now a synthetic version available that smells almost exactly like the real thing but doesn't involve the slaughter of the animal. That is a fine development for fragrances; however, when it comes to aromatherapy, merely smelling like the real thing isn't good enough. Science isn't even close to being able to replicate the molecular makeup of a complete essential oil in the laboratory. Essential oils are highly complex substances with many different components. Most essential oils have about 100 constituents, but some have more. For example, eucalyptus has about 250 and rose has approximately 260. All biological entities comprise chemicals that can be broken down, but an organic substance such as eucalyptol, which is the chief constituent in eucalyptus oil, acts much more effectively as an antiseptic when it's working within the structure of the essential oil than when it is chemically isolated and combined with other synthetic ingredients. Although science has been able to isolate the active ingredients in many plants and has used them effectively to make medicines (about 25 percent of today's drugs contain active ingredients synthesized from plants), often they have brutal side effects. While essential oils are powerful medicines, when used in the correct doses they rarely have side effects and their actions mostly work synergistically with the rest of the body.

This principle of synergism is very important to the understanding of aromatherapy as an art and science. When two things work synergistically, their combined power is greater than the sum of their individual actions. The ingredients of essential oils, many of which are still a mystery to science, heal in harmony. This explains why synthetic equivalents—which are never whole and contain only what scientists deduce are the active ingredients—do not always heal in harmony and certainly do not impact upon the subtle energies of the body. Synthetic compounds are fine for perfume, but dedicated aromatherapists would never use laboratory-made chemicals in therapeutic practices. Believing that nature is a better chemist than humans, aromatherapists employ the living technology of plants, contained in pure essential oils, to treat the body. When it comes to healing, synthetic substances lack the "dynamism" and "intelligence" of nature. In other words, nature is smarter than us and her handiwork infinitely more complex, sophisticated, and elegant.

These pure, natural, living substances, the essences of plants and flowers, deliver health-giving messages to the body, mind, and spirit.

The real thing

Beware—the term "natural" is stamped everywhere by manufacturers of home and personal-care products seeking to cash in on the glamour of nature. If you want to benefit from true healing ingredients harvested directly from nature, read labels carefully. Don't be fooled by so-called "natural" products claiming to contain the bounty of nature but calling themselves "fragrance oils" or "perfume oils." The quality and price of essential oils depend on many factors— the country in which the plant was cultivated, the abundance of the plant, the climatic conditions the year the oil was cultivated, and how the plants are collected, stored, and processed. Like wines, essential oils have good and bad years. Many essential oils are expensive because large amounts of plant materials are needed to produce small amounts of oil. When purchasing essential oils, ask where the oil comes from and try to find some information on the supplier. Some essential oils, such as citrus oils, have a limited shelf life, so they need to be fresh. Oils must be stored in a dry, dark environment away from direct sunlight. The best way to buy pure essential oils is to sniff many different brands and varieties. It sounds trite, but the nose always knows, and with experience, you will be able to distinguish between pure, natural essential oils and synthetic fragrances or adulterated blends.

Essential oils are medicines. Although adverse reactions and allergies are very rare, these are powerful chemical cocktails that in the wrong doses can be toxic to the body.

As with any potent substance, great care must be taken when administering essential oils. In many countries essential oils are taken internally, but only as prescribed by a qualified practitioner. It is not advisable to ingest essential oils. None of the formulas or recipes in this book is designed to be taken internally. Here are a few points to remember when you prescribe essential oils for yourself, friends, and family.

1. Do not apply undiluted essential oils directly to the skin or mucous membranes.

2. The following oils have been known to cause skin irritations if used directly on the skin and absorbed in very high concentrations. Make sure you use at least $1^1/_2$ fl oz of carrier oil to 2 drops of these oils and no more than 1 drop in bath water (In aromatherapy a carrier is any substance that will deliver essential oils to the body. Cold-pressed vegetable oils are most often used to carry essential oils for use on the face or body. Carrier oils dilute essential oils, making stronger oils safe to use on the skin.) Cinnamon Bark, Cinnamon Leaf, Bay, Clove Leaf, Clove Bud, Pimento, Red Thyme, Lemongrass, Peppermint, Savory, Oregano.

3. Always keep out of reach of children.

4. When preparing massage oils for children up to six years of age, don't use more than 8 drops of a mild essential oil to $1^1/_2$ fl oz of a carrier oil. For children between six and twelve, use no more than 10 drops per $1^1/_2$ fl oz of carrier oil. Always dilute essential oils in a carrier oil before dropping them into a child's bath. Never use more than 3 drops for children between birth and six years, or more than 6 drops for children between six and twelve years of age.

5. Avoid using any known irritant oils in baths.

6. There are thirty oils listed in this chapter. Of those, the essential oils that should not be used by pregnant women and nursing mothers have been noted under the "Safe Use" listing. However, there are some oils not covered by the list that should be avoided by pregnant women: Armoise, Camphor, Cypriol, Davana, Hyssop, Pennyroyal, Birch, Tarragon. General care should be taken with these oils (to be used in minute dilutions): Anise, Basil, Bay, Clary Sage, Clove Leaf, Clove Bud, Fennel, Myrrh, Nutmeg, Pimento Berry, Rosemary, Altas Cedar, Red Thyme, Spearmint, Savory, Oregano.

7. Essential oils work beautifully and economically in the treatment of many common physiological and psychological conditions, but they should not replace the advice of a qualified doctor or holistic therapist.

8. Do not use essential oils in place of medications prescribed by a physician.

9. When you first use a new essential oil blend, perform a patch test. Apply a couple of drops of the essential oil with a base/carrier oil to the inside forearm and wait for any reaction to occur. Reactions are unusual, but any redness and irritation is mostly likely to develop within a few minutes or hours of application.

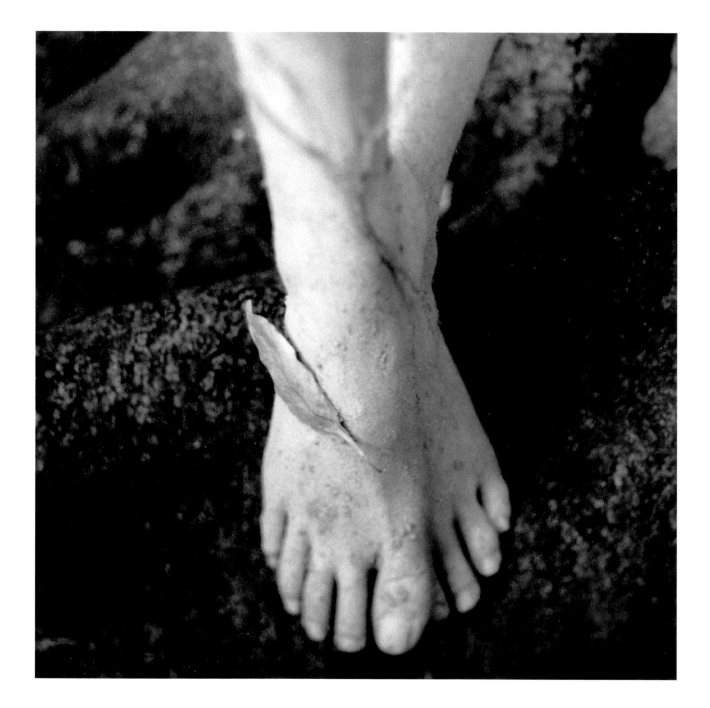

There are hundreds
of essential oils on the market
today. The thirty oils listed here are
generally easy to obtain and widely used
in aromatherapy. All these oils have
a proven track record and impart their own
particular healing magic. Essential oils
represent the individual character of
the plant from which they are derived, the
complex, eccentric, wonderful, bewitching, exotic,
exciting world of nature. Some oils will surprise and
delight you, transporting you to an unexplored universe of
sensual pleasure. Some will simply not appeal to you.
One thing is certain: Finding the right oils for you
will take you on an exquisite journey into the
art and science of aromatherapy.

History gave basil a bad rap. When the herb was introduced into Europe, it spooked people. All sorts of stories and bad PR surrounded it. One funky tale tells of a man who smelled basil so often it bred a scorpion in his head. It was also thought in ancient times that priests might be able to create scorpions by crushing basil between two stones. Perhaps this arose because the name *basilicum* comes from two words, the Greek *basilicos* which means "royal" and the Latin *basiliscus*, which refers to a serpent. However, basil was reported to cure scorpion stings and other insect bites. In India basil was always associated with funeral practices. In the West Indies, they have a better slant on basil—when soaked in water and sprinkled around shops it's supposed to attract business and good luck. Aromatherapists say basil helps promote higher states of awareness and open the heart and mind. Because of its hormonelike actions, basil is said to help reduce impotence and infertility, and increase sexual interest. Interestingly, the astrological sign Scorpio is associated with the sex life and reproductive organs. With basil's connection with crawly critters that sting, it's not surprising that it's said to put the zing back into your sex life. *Benefits:* Basil is great in a crisis. It has an extraordinary antispasmodic action that makes it useful in the treatment of muscular cramps, all respiratory tract infections, asthma, and bronchitis. The oil possesses antiviral, anti-infectious, antivenin and antibacterial properties. Basil loves to clean up ulcers, bites, weepy acne, and intestinal cramps, and works like a dream on wounds. This oil is uplifting and stimulating and helps get rid of the blues. *Safe use:* Infused into the air and in small amounts in massage and bath blends, basil stimulates the nervous system, relieves fevers and digestive disorders. *Caution:* There is some evidence that this oil can bring on labor in the latter stages of pregnancy and it is also known to increase milk supply in nursing mothers. Basil has been known to be toxic when taken internally.

Common name: Basil (sweet)
Botanical name: Ocimum basilicum
Essence from: Flowering tops and leaves of herb
Cultivated in: Comoros, Madagascar, Vietnam, West Australia, India
Aroma: Sweet and spicy
Perfume note: Top

Bergamot has a romantic history. Christopher Columbus was reported to have found the tree in the Canary Islands and introduced it to Italy and Spain. Its name is derived from Bergamo, where the tree was first cultivated. Bergamot has been known to induce blissful sleep and has a cooling and refreshing quality that helps quell nervous emotions and frustration. One of the most common ingredients in perfumery, bergamot is responsible for the aromatic taste of Earl Grey tea. *Benefits:* Bergamot goes straight to the heart. This uplifting and vibrant oil helps relieve stress, depression, and fatigue. Bergamot is used as a calmative to help soothe breathing difficulties, respiratory infections, and lung diseases. As a natural deodorant, bergamot will neutralize foul smells and bring harmony to the environment. Bergamot is also an effective digestive and helps relieve the problems associated with dyspepsia, flatulence, colic, and hiccups.

Common name: Bergamot
Botanical name: Citrus bergamia
Essence from: Peel of nearly ripe fruit
Cultivated in: Italy, Morocco
Aroma: Rich and sweet, with floral undertones
Perfume note: Top

Bergamot is also useful in the treatment of oily skin, acne, seborrhea, and wounds. *Safe use:* Bergamot blends with almost every essential oil and is safe to use in massage, baths, infusions, burners, and perfumes. Used as a mild skin tonic, bergamot will balance skin and heal blemishes. *Caution:* Bergamot must be diluted when used on the skin, as it can cause irritations in high doses. Bergamot has photosensitizing properties (which makes the skin more sensitive to UV light); therefore this oil can promote sunburn, and sunbathing should be avoided after significant use for up to twelve hours.

Cedarwood may have been one of the first essential oils ever made. Used lavishly in cosmetics, in mummification practices, and as an insect repellent, the Egyptians prized the oil so highly they annexed the great Lebanese forests to ensure a plentiful supply. The Native Americans considered the *Juniperus virginiana* cedar to be sacred. They believed the Great Spirit who created the universe left a special mark on all plants capable of healing people—a pointed top. According to legend, when the creator of all things made the cedar tree, Grandmother Earth loved it so much that she filled its center with blood, turning the inside red. The Native Americans discovered that when the wood was burned and inhaled it cleared the sinuses, relaxed the larynx, and soothed the soul. *Benefits:* Cedarwood is a potent cleanser. It combats acne and both excessively dry or oily scalps. As an insect repellent, cedarwood acts quickly and effectively and will also treat an insect sting or itch. Dermatitis, eczema, and psoriasis are no match for the efficient cedarwood when it's diffused into the skin. When infused into the atmosphere, cedarwood will treat upper respiratory tract infections, clear the sinuses, and help heal nervous conditions. Cedarwood gives a whiff of the forest, which brings balance and peace to stressed-out city slickers. *Safe use:* Cedarwood in high doses will irritate the skin, so it is advisable to use only a maximum of 2 drops if you want to bathe with this oil. However, diluted in a carrier and mixed with other oils, it will work wonders on acne and other skin problems. When it's released into the atmosphere it works as a nerve sedative and eases mental tension. *Caution:* Cedarwood is not to be used on infants or on women during pregnancy.

Common name: Cedarwood (Altas)
Botanical name: Cedrus atlantica
Essence from: Wood of the tree
Cultivated in: North Africa
Aroma: Dry, woody, strong
Perfume note: Base

Common name: German Chamomile
Botanical name: Matricaria recruita
Essence from: The dried flowers of the herb
Cultivated in: Hungary, Egypt
Aroma: Herbaceous, sweet, warm, and rich
Perfume note: Middle

Chamomile comes from the Greek word *chamaimelon* or "earth apple," which seems an apt description of its scent. The ancient Egyptians dedicated the flower to the sun because of its ability to cure fever. German chamomile is often brewed as a sedative tea and is widely regarded as a calmative and digestive. Chamomile has been used for centuries in herbal medicine as a cure for insomnia and anxiety. Roman chamomile is more sedative than German chamomile and when used together on skin conditions they can produce powerful results. *Benefits:* Chamomile has a reputation for putting people to sleep but that is the least of its powers. Chamomile has remarkable anti-inflammatory and antibacterial powers. The oil is purifying, soothing, calming, and restorative. It has the ability to increase the production of white corpuscles, which aids healing and boosts the immune system. When used in conjunction with massage it can effectively treat gout and rheumatism. Chamomile has been used for centuries to treat neuralgia, teething in children, some of the symptoms of menopause, migraine, and all gastric and intestinal problems. On wounds, herpes, eczema, and any skin irritation, chamomile soothes and heals quickly. *Safe use:* When used in burners and steam baths chamomile has the ability to clear the air and relax fraught nerves. As a poultice on open wounds and sores like herpes, it has mild nerve sedative properties. Chamomile doesn't like water—it clots and clings to the sides of the tub. However, mixed with other oils, such as lavender, and dropped in the bath, chamomile will help heal irritated skin and relax the entire body before bed. Chamomile is safe to use in massage on children and pregnant women.

66

At many stages in history, cinnamon was as precious as gold. The innocent, unobtrusive bark flavored the food of Europe, was dropped into the medications of the Chinese Emperor Shen Nung, perfumed Cleopatra's potions, and has since turned up in sweet buns and treats—even Coca-cola has a hint of this precious spice. Cinnamon has always been

Common name: Cinnamon Bark
Botanical name: Cinnamomum zeylanicum
Essence from: Inner bark of shoots from cultivated, coppiced trees and dried flower buds of tropical trees
Cultivated in: Sri Lanka, Madagascar, Southern India, West Indies, Islands of the Seychelles
Aroma: Warm and spicy, sweet
Perfume note: Middle/base

associated with money and trade and is said to increase abundance, both spiritual and financial. Its connection with food accounts for its comforting, familiar aroma. *Benefits:* Cinnamon has an alluring, spicy aroma that is nothing short of mouthwatering. In massage and baths cinnamon helps stimulate digestion, circulation, and respiration. It is often prescribed as a heart tonic because it stimulates cardiac activity. The oil has mild antispasmodic properties and helps speed elimination in the body. Cinnamon has been reported to kill the typhoid bacillus and is regarded as a strong antiseptic. The oil has an effect on the hormones, and aromatherapists often use it to help regulate menstrual cycles and boost the sexual urge. Cinnamon has also been reported to help treat stings and insect bites. *Safe use:* When infused into the atmosphere, cinnamon will relieve melancholia and boost psychic awareness. The oil treats infection and makes an effective inhalation. It is often used in cooking and cough elixirs, but when used in an essential oil form can be very potent. *Caution:* Cinnamon can irritate the skin, so it should not be used at all in baths and diluted to no more than $\frac{1}{2}$ percent in massage preparations. Do not apply undiluted cinnamon to the skin or mucous membranes.

Common name: Clary Sage
Botanical name: Salvia sclarea
Essence from: Herb and flowers
Cultivated in: France, India, New Zealand, America
Aroma: Herbaceous and floral
Perfume note: Top

The name "clary sage" is derived from the Latin *clarus*, or "clear," probably because the seeds were once used to clear foreign particles from the eyes. The plant played an important role in herbal medicine in bygone days and was used as a poultice on stings and bites. Clary sage is most famous for its ability to bring on states of euphoria and can have narcoticlike effects. According to a seventeenth-century writer, it was used in England to "sophisticate beer"—which meant that those who drank the intoxicating elixir were sent into heady, drunken spins and after much "insane exhilaration" were found the morning after with a hangover to end all hangovers. There is some evidence that the herb releases adrenaline, which accounts for its ability to lift depression and power the sex drive. *Benefits:* Clary sage is one of nature's best beauty aids. It has a profound effect on the skin and its antiseptic action can help kill skin fungus and treat dandruff. Clary sage will reduce inflammation of the skin and is said to help diminish wrinkles. As a treatment for dry and aging skin it will soothe and help restore tone. Clary sage also has an estrogenlike action, which helps regulate menstrual cycles, reduce PMS, control many premenopausal symptoms, and reduce period pain. It can also encourage labor and aid delivery. This uplifting oil performs well as a deodorant and has a calming effect on the nervous system. *Safe use:* Clary sage is related to common sage, but the two essential oils have quite different actions. Clary sage is commonly used in potpourri and as a fixative when blending aromas. It can be applied in a poultice for muscle strains and as a tonic for dry skin. The oil is said to bring on states of euphoria when inhaled or in massage and bath combinations. *Caution:* During pregnancy the use of clary sage should be monitored by a qualified aromatherapist. The combination of clary and alcohol can produce nightmares and nausea and large doses can induce headaches.

Common name: Clove Bud
Botanical name: Eugenia caryophyllus
Essence from: Dried flower buds
Cultivated in: Madagascar, West Indies, Zanzibar
Aroma: Distinct, refreshing, sweet, spicy
Perfume note: Middle

Clove, along with cinnamon, was a valuable commodity in the ancient world. Clove found its way into teas and tinctures, poultices and pomanders. It was a widely used medicine and an early anesthetic and antiseptic. Clove was very expensive and its distinctive taste was much admired in liqueurs and other aromatic beverages. In the old days, pomanders were made of oranges studded with cloves to ward off infectious diseases. Clove essence is one of the ingredients of Koheul, an ophthalmic ointment used by the Arabs. In the not-so-distant past the Germans developed a clove-based general anesthetic. The drug eliminates the need for a "pre-med" injection and allows the patient to regain consciousness shortly after the anesthetic is administered. Some say clove has similar properties to opium, which perhaps explains its wide use in perfumery and its fame as an aphrodisiac. *Benefits:* Clove is the dentist's best friend. Well known for its strong antiseptic properties, it is widely used in dentistry to numb and protect the gums and nerves. Clove is used as a general stimulant and will revive the mind and stimulate the nervous system. Massaged into the abdomen, the oil is a great gastric calmative and relieves spasmodic pain from dyspepsia, diarrhea, and flatulence. Dabbed on wounds, leg ulcers, and mosquito bites, clove will quickly clear skin infections. Rubbed into the wood in a wardrobe, clove will repel moths. *Safe use:* Clove is said to make a great analgesic and when used as a compress on sore teeth or ulcers will act with mercurial speed. When infused into the atmosphere, clove will brighten the spirits and restore balance to the mind. Clove is also a good insect repellent and can be applied in minimal, diluted doses to the skin to heal open sores. *Caution:* Pregnant women and children should avoid this oil. Clove bud is not suggested for bath preparations.

Eu and *kalypto*
are derived from the Greek
words for "well" and "cover," which
refer to the covered stamens of the eucalyptus
tree. The Australian Aborigines called it "Kino,"
and often bound the leaves around wounds to heal
them. A concoction called "Sydney Peppermint," an
oil extracted from the eucalyptus leaves, was
exported to England as a digestive tonic in
the early days of the colony. *Benefits:* When
it comes to killing germs, eucalyptus has
muscle. It is a powerful general antiseptic
and works particularly well on the upper
respiratory tract when inhaled—treating bronchitis, influenza,
pulmonary tuberculosis, and asthma. Fevers due to infection, the pain of
rheumatism, neuralgia, and migraine have all been known to subside when
eucalyptus is lovingly massaged into the skin of sufferers. And it can ward off
airborne disease and insects when it is burned. *Safe use:* Eucalyptus comes into its
own as a disinfectant. Either infused into the atmosphere or rubbed onto surfaces,
this oil will keep germs at bay. Safe for use in compresses, poultices, and massage
blends, eucalyptus speeds the healing of wounds, infections, acne, and sores. Massaged
into the chest, it will help patients overcome flu, coughs, and colds. Eucalyptus
has a cooling, refreshing effect on the emotions and helps clear the head
and aid concentration. *Caution:* High doses of eucalyptus can
be toxic: Make sure you use the correct doses
when prescribing.

Common name: Eucalyptus australiana
Botanical name: Eucalyptus radiata
Essence from: Leaves
Cultivated in: Australia
Aroma: Strong, fresh, citruslike with herbaceous undertones
Perfume note: Top

Common name: Fennel (sweet)
Botanical name: Foeniculum vulgare
Essence from: Roots, seeds, leaves
Cultivated in: Mediterranean, Central Europe, India, Japan, New Zealand, Australia, America
Aroma: Sweet, fresh, reminiscent of aniseed
Perfume note: Middle

Roman
soldiers chewed fennel seeds on
long marches to keep hunger at bay. The
ancient Chinese used fennel for its diuretic properties
and as a slimming agent. The ancient Greeks wove fennel into
chaplets and used them to crown victorious athletes. Fennel had religious and
ceremonial significance in Greek, Hindu, and Chinese traditions. *Benefits:* Fennel
is famous for its ability to fight fat and reduce cellulite. The herb has a
reputation for suppressing the appetite, and it has diuretic properties that
help prevent fluid retention and speed the elimination of toxins from
the body. The essential oil is commonly used as a digestive and to
relieve colitis, constipation, flatulence, and indigestion. Fennel
has been used to treat urinary tract infections and kidney stones, as well as weak eyesight because it
helps stimulate the liver (in Chinese medicine, the eyes are related to the liver through energy
meridians). Fennel has a powerful effect on the hormones and can help regulate scanty
menstruation. On a metaphysical level, fennel is said to increase one's life span, boost
confidence, and inspire courage. *Safe use:* In very high doses fennel causes
convulsions, but applied locally in moderation, it can help bruises,
indigestion, and sore gums. When infused into the air it is said to
repel psychic vampires who drain your energy. Many
aromatherapists suggest not using this oil at all during
pregnancy and do not prescribe it for people with
epilepsy or psychotic illnesses.

Frankincense has been used in ceremonial and religious rites for more than 5,000 years. You could count on it being at every party. It was the most prized and costly temple accessory in the ancient world. The name is derived from medieval French for "luxurious incense," which comes from the original name Olbanum, or "Oil from Lebanon." The valuable herb was supposedly one of the gifts given to the baby Jesus. It was imported from Egypt and Africa many thousands of years ago and was immediately taken up as a perfume and used in cosmetics and medicine. *Benefits:* Frankincense has staying power. When they opened King Tut's tomb in 1926 the scent, captured in tiny vials, was still clinging to life, more than 3,000 years after its use-by date. Frankincense has a profound effect on the mucous membranes and is one of the most valuable oils for the treatment of respiratory infections. It speeds up the healing process of persistent wounds and promotes the formation of scar tissue. The oil has an affinity with the urino-genital tract and can relieve cystitis and heavy periods. Safely used during pregnancy and childbirth, its calming action can soothe labor pains. Frankincense has a tonifying effect and is renowned for its anti-aging properties and action on dry and oily skin conditions. Frankincense is a powerful anti-depressant and has been known to pacify bad tempers. It has also been used as an aid to meditation for many centuries and is said to liberate the spirit. *Safe use:* Frankincense is generally safe to use in massage oils, bath blends, and in burners to deepen inhalation. It is an excellent skin tonic and can be used in cosmetic preparations.

Common name: Frankincense
Botanical name: Boswellia carterii
Essence from: Resin from the bark of the tree
Cultivated in: North Africa, Middle East
Aroma: Woody, spicy, deep
Perfume note: Base

70

Common name: Geranium
Botanical name: Pelargonium asperum/gravolens
Essence from: Aerial plant parts
Cultivated in: Comoros, Egypt, China, Morocco
Aroma: Floral, leafy, fresh, herbaceous
Perfume note: Middle

Geranium (abundant in folklore) was once hailed as a great heal-all. Native Americans used the plant to cure a range of ailments, from toothache to cholera to neuralgia, gonorrhea, and ulcers. Throughout the centuries, people would plant geranium around their cottages to keep evil spirits at bay. Islamic myth contends that geranium is a gift from Allah because its smell is sublime and its actions profound. The French began commercial production of geranium oil in the nineteenth century, and its popularity is undiminished today. *Benefits:* Geranium has played healer in cultures of ancient civilizations too numerous to count. A potent healing plant, geranium has been used to treat tumors, cholera, and bone fractures. It is a powerful antispasmodic and has been known to help regulate the hormones. When rubbed into the skin, geranium helps digestive upsets, infections, neuralgia, PMS, and varicose veins and promotes wound healing. It is well regarded as a lymphotonic and acts powerfully on skin fungus and other growths. Geranium is widely used in perfume because its divine aroma is calming, balancing, and uplifting. *Safe use:* Geranium is often recommended to treat skin problems because it helps heal wounds. Aromatherapists may prescribe the oil during pregnancy since it has virtually no contraindications.

The origins of grapefruit are not easily tracked down. It was apparently first sighted in Asia and was reported to be a hybrid of orange, although its sometimes bitter taste is more reminiscent of the tangy lemon. Most often found on the breakfast table covered in a crystal cloak of sugar, grapefruit is also popular as an ingredient in perfumery.

Benefits: Grapefruit is a great reviver. This uplifting oil stimulates the appetite, the mind, and the vascular system. Grapefruit is a pick-me-up when the woes of the world start knocking at the door. It acts as an antiseptic, disinfectant, diuretic, and general stimulant. As a skin and hair treatment, grapefruit will stimulate microcirculation within the skin, and bring radiance and tone. Grapefruit has also been known to chase away fatigue and beat jet lag.

Safe use: Grapefruit has mild photosensitizing properties (as do all the citrus essential oils) and has been known to accelerate tanning. Avoid direct sunlight for up to twelve hours when you have grapefruit on your skin. Grapefruit is also slightly astringent, and while it works well in hair tonics and footbaths, it is not to be used in baths.

Common name: Grapefruit
Botanical name: Citrus paradisi
Essence from: Skin of the fruit
Cultivated in: Australia, Brazil, America, Israel
Aroma: Sweet, citrus, fruity, sharp, refreshing
Perfume note: Top

Common name: Jasmine
Botanical name: Jasminum grandiflorum/Jasminum officinale
Essence from: Flowers picked straight from the vines at night
Cultivated in: Algeria, Morocco, France, China, Turkey, Italy, Egypt
Aroma: Exotic, rich, sweet, floral
Perfume note: Base

Jasmine has earned its place in history as the "king of flowers" next to rose, "the queen," because its fragrance is redolent of forbidden sex in moonlit, blooming gardens. In India it is known as "Queen of the Night," and symbolizes divine hope. In China jasmine finds its way into tea and ointments, and the Chinese believe it symbolizes the sweetness of woman. One fl oz of Jean Patou's famous fragrance Joy is said to contain 10,600 crushed flowers, and for this reason Joy is one of the costliest and most coveted fragrances in the world today. *Benefits:* Jasmine spreads good vibes as soon as the nose detects its delicious scent. This oil can turn an ardent pessimist into an optimist with one whiff. To add to its list of charms, jasmine helps regulate the female reproductive system and relieve PMS, menstrual pain, and spotting—good news for the husbands and lovers of pre-menstrual women. The oil is warm and seductive and has been used as an aphrodisiac since Eve wooed Adam. When applied to the skin, jasmine is beneficial for dry skin, stretch marks, joint pains, and dermatitis. On a more subtle level, jasmine is said to stimulate the creative urge, inspiring artists to paint, dance, sculpt, and write. Jasmine also unearths deep emotions such as compassion and confidence. *Safe use:* As a perfume jasmine has few rivals. When it's released into the atmosphere virgins are in danger. Dropped into a bath, jasmine has the ability to turn a gray day into a carnival, but it must be used moderately. As with all precious things, less is often more. *Caution:* Overdosing on jasmine can cause absent-mindedness and irritated skin. Jasmine is generally a very safe oil and at usual doses has no ill effects. It is not generally used during pregnancy because it can help induce uterine contractions; however, when massaged into the feet, hands, and head during labor, it helps with birth.

In Egypt juniper oil was used in the embalming process and the berries were used as a digestive. In China and Tibet juniper was used to help prevent the spread of infectious diseases. The oil has been used to ward off evil spirits, purify, and cleanse for many centuries. European herbalists used juniper as an integral part of their healing repertoire. Juniper was known to treat hemorrhoids, and as the basis of gin, has visited and left some dubious watering holes. Curiously, juniper imparts the scent of violets to urine. *Benefits:* Juniper sends germs packing. Massaged into the body or infused in baths, juniper is a good antiseptic and aids the digestive tract and respiratory system. Juniper is said to have defeated even the most worthy foes—cholera, dysentery, and typhoid. Juniper generates heat: When massaged into the skin it makes the body sweat, warms the skin, and heats the gut. As a treatment for cold hands and feet, juniper dropped into socks or gloves will help prevent chilblains. Juniper promotes the formation of scar tissue and acts as a diuretic. Diluted, juniper will help rid cats and dogs of fleas and speed the recovery of wounds. Juniper also fortifies and cleanses the mind. *Safe use:* Although juniper makes a terrific diuretic and can help prevent kidney stones, too much can overload the kidneys. *Caution:* Juniper should be avoided during pregnancy and is not suitable for infants or babies.

Common name: Juniper
Botanical name: Juniperus communis
Essence from: Berries and sometimes berry laden branches of the tree
Cultivated in: Grows wild all over Africa, Asia, Czechoslovakia, Germany, Italy, North America, Scandinavia
Aroma: Rich, balsamic, fresh and woody-sweet
Perfume note: Middle

The lavender plant was probably introduced to England by the Romans, who used it for bathing. The name lavender is derived from the Latin word *lavare*, "to wash," hinting at lavender's supreme anti-infectious ability. The ancient Greeks, Romans, and Persians all burned lavender to ward off the epidemics that frequently swept through their communities. Later, lavender was used in Europe to disinfect nasty wounds and treat ailments brought on by various plagues. Lavender's main claim to fame is that the famous French chemist, Gattefossé, discovered its marvelous ability to heal when he burned his hand in a laboratory and instinctively plunged it into a vat of lavender. The folklore associated with lavender tells of its magical ability to promote states of love and ecstasy. In North Africa women used this plant to guard against maltreatment by their husbands, and the scent is said to tame wild lions and tigers. *Benefits:* The handyman of any essential oil kit, lavender is kind to everyone and fixes just about anything. Purifying and calming, it enhances all skin types and restores mental balance. Lavender is commonly used to treat bites and stings, burns, eczema/dermatitis, insomnia, nervous tension, lice, asthma, bruises, and colds and flu. It is also a highly effective anti-inflammatory agent and helps reduce the pain associated with muscular cramps, menstrual pain, and rasping coughs. The oil also has a mild antibiotic and decongestant action and will speed recovery from upper respiratory tract infections when it's inhaled. It is one of the mildest essential oils, but its actions can be profound. Lavender is one of the few essential oils that can be applied directly to the skin, and when dabbed right onto a superficial burn, the oil's dramatic ability to stimulate the healing process takes immediate effect. With its ability to neutralize toxins, lavender soothes minor insect bites and stings. Used regularly in face washes and baths, lavender has a calming, restorative effect on the skin. The antibacterial properties keep infections at bay. The oil has been known to cure headaches, reduce fevers, and modify stress. Much, much more than granny's fragrant toilet water, lavender deserves a place in any bathroom cabinet. *Safe use:* For use in poultices, skin tonics, baths, fragrant oil for burning, and a perfect addition to any massage blend.

Common name: True Lavender
Botanical name: Lavandula angustifolia
Essence from: Flowering tops and leaves
Cultivated in: Bulgaria, France, Tasmania, Hungary, Spain
Aroma: Herbaceous and floral
Perfume note: Middle/top

Lemon juice is so versatile it will even clean silver. Lemon dissolves rust spots on fine white linen and removes ink from writers' fingers. Lemon oil repels moths and ants, so it's a handy essence to sprinkle into wardrobes and cupboards. The name comes from the Arabic *laimun* and the Persian *limun*, referring to citrus fruits. The Egyptians used it as an antidote to food poisoning and viral epidemics, and discovered that the juice and the rind worked efficiently as a contraceptive aid. *Caution:* Don't try this method at home! *Benefits:* Lemon is one of the hardest working of all essential oils. It makes a superior digestive aid and a potent antiseptic. Lemon will defeat the tuberculosis bacillus in twenty minutes and the juice will demolish 92 percent of all bacteria in oysters within fifteen minutes. Applied to the skin, lemon essence will keep bacteria and infections at bay, and inhaled into the lungs, will clear persistent infections. Lemon is said to banish wrinkles and put restless ulcers to bed. It can be applied to herpes, chilblains, boils, acne, and insect bites, and inhaled to treat the flu, migraines, and nosebleeds. Lemon lowers blood pressure, promotes the formation of scar tissue, and acts as an antirheumatic by relieving pain. It can also alleviate tension and refresh tired minds. *Safe use:* Released into the air, lemon purifies and kills lurking germs. As a bath companion, lemon is stimulating, uplifting, and exciting. In massage, lemon will treat a multitude of ills. *Caution:* It has photosensitizing properties and thus can accelerate sunburn.

Common name: Lemon
Botanical name: Citrus limon
Essence from: Rind of the fruit
Cultivated in: Australia, America, Italy, Israel, Spain, Portugal
Aroma: Fresh, sharp, citrus, stimulating
Perfume note: Top

Lemongrass has been used in Asian, Mexican, and South American cooking for thousands of years. The herb has been used in primitive rituals for purification and to promote psychic awareness. *Benefits:* Lemongrass has get-up-and-go, driving the nervous system and stimulating the internal plumbing. Massaged into the belly, lemongrass acts as a digestive stimulant and powerful anti-inflammatory. Lemongrass will get rid of fungal infections and tone the skin. The oil has been known to stimulate the flow of milk in nursing mothers. As a booster on days when the engine stops short, lemongrass is a great pick-me-up. Ironically, in very small doses, less than $1/2$ percent dilution, lemongrass will sedate the mind and nervous system. *Safe use:* Lemongrass can be quite strong when in direct contract with the skin, and must be diluted (2–3 drops maximum for any formula) if applied to the body. Infused into the air, lemongrass strengthens the emotions and clears the atmosphere. *Caution:* Don't use in the bath.

Common name: Lemongrass
Botanical name: Cymbopogon citratus
Essence from: Leaves of the plant
Cultivated in: India, Madagascar, the Antilles
Aroma: Sweet, strong, lemony
Perfume note: Top

The name is
derived from the Greek word
margaron, meaning "pearl." The word
origanum is derived from two Greek words, *oros*,
meaning "mountain," and *ganos*, meaning "joy." The Greeks
used the herb for medicines as well as cosmetics. It was used to
treat dropsy, narcotic poisoning, and convulsions. The herb was planted
in graveyards to ward off evil spirits and given to newlyweds to give them luck.
Legend has it the goddess Venus gave marjoram its sweet fragrance. Because it
both relaxes and expands, many professional singers have used an infusion of marjoram
sweetened with honey to help tune their throat and vocal cords. *Benefits:* Marjoram puts out
fires. Whether it's the burning pain of rheumatism or the fire that burns in the darker realms
of the psyche, marjoram's ability to ease and comfort are second to none. Marjoram has been
known to reduce the cramps associated with menstruation, and the pain of migraines, constipation,
and indigestion. The oil makes a sublime expectorant, expelling mucus from the lungs, and can
help relieve the symptoms of asthma, bronchitis, colds, and sore throats. Marjoram has a relaxing
effect on muscle strains and can relieve the symptoms of seasickness. *Safe use:* In a compress
applied to any ache, marjoram is nurturing and sedating, but in large amounts marjoram is
stupefying. When high levels of physical performance
are required, marjoram is a poor companion. *Caution:*
The oil is not recommended for people with low blood
pressure. It is known to be an anti-aphrodisiac
and can take the excitement out of the most
potent advances. This oil is not suitable
for use during pregnancy. Marjoram
is also not recommended for
people who suffer from
depression.

Common name: Marjoram (sweet)
Botanical name: Origanum marjorana
Essence from: The flowers
Cultivated in: Yugoslavia, Iran,
Hungary, Egypt, France
Aroma: Warm, rich, slightly spicy
Perfume note: Base

Common name: Myrrh
Botanical name: Commiphora molmol
Essence from: Resin from the branches
Cultivated in: Middle East, Somalia, Asia
Aroma: Cloudy, musky, balsamic, gumlike
Perfume note: Base

Myrrh is as old as time itself. It is thought (although it is too long ago now to really know), that the word myrrh is derived from the Hebrew *mar*, which means "bitter." The essence was used in incense, perfumes, cosmetics, and medicines all over the ancient world. The Greeks used myrrh on the battlefield to treat wounds and reduce inflammations. The Egyptians burned myrrh every day as part of their offerings to the sun god. Myrrh was known as a good remedy for herpes and as a superior cosmetic—a recipe for a facial mask using myrrh was found on the Ebers papyrus dating from the eighteenth Egyptian dynasty (1580 B.C.). According to Greek legend, it originated from the tears of Myrrha, a daughter of the King of Cypress, who had been changed into a plant. *Benefits:* Myrrh doesn't drag its heels when there's work to be done. It will clear up the most persistent boils and wounds, eczema, skin ulcers, bed sores, and athlete's foot. Myrrh is principally an anti-inflammatory, a healing and antiseptic oil. As an expectorant, myrrh banishes mucus lurking in the lungs and clears any upper respiratory tract infection. Rubbed over the belly, myrrh will fortify weak stomachs, stimulate the appetite, and help treat diarrhea and flatulence. This oil is said to cool heated emotions, promote courage, and bring balance to the mind. *Safe use:* Diluted in a poultice or compress on a wound, myrrh works quickly to disinfect and heal. Infused into the air, myrrh will harmonize fraught nerves. *Caution:* It should be avoided during pregnancy.

Common name: Neroli
Botanical name: Citrus aurantium
Essence from: Flowers of the bitter orange tree
Cultivated in: France, Italy, America
Aroma: Sweet, floral, citrus
Perfume note: Base

Neroli is made from the flowers of the bitter orange tree. Orange blossoms have been used for centuries in Chinese medicine and cosmetics. The flowers symbolize innocence and love in many folkloric traditions and are often used in European wedding rituals. Neroli takes its name from a sixteenth-century Italian princess, Nerola, who used the flowers to perfume her bathwater and clothes. Orange water has been a popular ingredient in perfumery for centuries, and is still used in the cuisine of Eastern European countries. *Benefits:* Neroli can make your heart sing. It has a calming effect on the cardiovascular system and can stop palpitations and anxiety attacks. This oil also has a rejuvenating action on the skin, improving elasticity, and helping to diminish scars, stretch marks, and broken veins. *Safe use:* Neroli has the power to bring even the most stressed out executives to a quiet state of mind—so perhaps it is not advisable to use this before making a big business deal. However, it relieves grief and can make a strong tranquilizer. Dropped into a bath or burner, neroli will cleanse the atmosphere and bring peace and harmony.

Common name: Orange
Botanical name:
Citrus sinensis
Essence from: Outer
peel of the fruit
Cultivated in: America,
Australia, Israel, India
Aroma: Refreshing,
sweet, citrus, warm
Perfume note: Top

The zippy, tangy smell of orange is universally loved. The fragrance has been used in cosmetics and perfumes for eons. The name is thought to be derived from the Arabic *narandj,* and it is believed that the fruit was brought to Europe during the Crusades. In Greek mythology oranges were the "golden apples" brought into the Garden of Hesperides. *Benefits:* Orange is a big mover and shaker. Sluggish digestion and infection are no match for this big gun. Orange supports tissue regeneration and as a total body tonic orange is stimulating and rejuvenating. It is a good antiseptic and treats mouth ulcers and any slowly healing sore. As a treatment for poor circulation, fluid retention, and cellulite, orange is said to work like a dream. Orange will pep up the emotions and promote open communication. *Safe use:* Orange can be excitable, so watch out for its bite in high doses. *Caution:* Orange can also be irritating, so it must be diluted if used in the bath or on the skin. Orange has photosensitizing properties and can accelerate sunburn.

In the traditional medical systems of China, India, Japan, and Malaysia, patchouli has played a starring role. It was a tonic for snake bites and insect stings and was taken as a general body tonic. In India patchouli was used to scent clothes and linen and has long been used in perfumery as a fixative. Patchouli blended with camphor gives Indian ink its characteristic aroma. Patchouli was brought to England in the late nineteenth century and was used in potpourris and scent sachets.

Patchouli, sandalwood, and jasmine—traditional Indian scents—were worn by the "flower children" of the 1960s.

Benefits: Patchouli instantly ignites the sexual flame. Long used as an aphrodisiac, patchouli can excite, delight, tantalize, and relax. Patchouli has many talents: antidepressant, antiseptic, and astringent. Patchouli is particularly valuable in skin care, as it relieves the pain of inflammation, speeds the healing of open wounds and the formation of scar tissue. Patchouli promotes psychic awareness and has the power to clarify thoughts. *Safe use:* Not everyone likes the musky, earthy scent of patchouli—redolent of armpits, wet earth, and burned wood, but it is safe to use as a perfume, and bath and massage aromatic.

Common name: Patchouli
Botanical name: Pogostemon patchouli
Essence from: The young leaves of the plant
Cultivated in: Malaysia, Indonesia, West Indies, South America
Aroma: Rich, earthy, exotic, musky
Perfume note: Base

There's an epic story about peppermint in Greek mythology. According to the story, Pluto was attracted to a young nymph, Mentha. Pluto's angry wife Persephone chased Mentha and when she caught her, trod her furiously into the ground. Pluto then turned Mentha into an herb. The herb peppermint has been used for centuries as a digestive and was found at ancient Greek and Roman feasts, its ability to settle the stomach giving it pride of place. The Hebrews used it for its aphrodisiac properties in perfumes and ointments. The essential oil of peppermint contains menthol, which can be used in inhalants and chewing mints. Peppermint is the most common flavoring in chewing gum, toothpaste, and breath fresheners. *Benefits:* Peppermint gets great PR wherever it goes. Used all over the world as a stimulant for the nervous system and a powerful digestive aid, peppermint is a potent tonic for the treatment of ulcers, irritable bowel syndrome, diarrhea, and flatulence. Its antiviral, anticatarrhal, and expectorant properties help speed recovery from colds, flu, and sinus congestion. Peppermint is an effective insect repellent and is a good treatment for many skin conditions like eczema, dermatitis, and ringworm. In small doses, peppermint can ease the itching of chicken pox. Massaged locally into affected areas, peppermint's antispasmodic action helps treat menstrual pain and sports injuries. Its anti-inflammatory action helps heal shingles, sciatica, neuralgia, and arthritis. Peppermint stimulates mental agility and helps concentration and memory. The oil can be very stimulating for the mind, relieving mental fatigue and depression. *Safe use:* Dropped into steam baths and burners, peppermint works quickly as a decongestant. Used in small amounts, it can purify and cleanse skin. *Caution:* This oil is not recommended for nursing mothers, as it can discourage milk flow. Great care must be taken in administering this oil—peppermint is generally stimulating, but if it is incorrectly used, it can often have a negative effect.

Common name: Peppermint
Botanical name: Mentha piperita
Essence from: Leaves
Cultivated in: Australia, America, Europe
Aroma: Strong, minty, sweet
Perfume note: Middle

The ancient Egyptians, Greeks, and Arabians used pine for its medicinal properties and noted it was useful in the treatment of lung infections. In 1534, Jacques Cartier learned from the Native Americans that extracts of pine cured and prevented scurvy, and the news of its powerful actions spread. As a common ingredient in soaps, disinfectants, and room deodorizers, pine is now a familiar smell in millions of bathrooms around the world. *Benefits:* Pine is a powerful antiseptic and decongestant, fighting disease and germs. Pine effectively treats chest and respiratory infections, and steam inhalations can help bronchitis, laryngitis, influenza, colds, catarrh, and sinusitis. The oil also has a stimulating effect on circulation, and can help relieve gout, sciatica, arthritis, and muscle strains. Pine has been used to treat urinary tract infections and gallstones. It stimulates the adrenal cortex, where a variety of steroids are produced, making it effective against impotence and depression. Pine boosts mental awareness and reduces fatigue. *Safe use:* Pine is a useful disinfectant that will diminish body odor when applied to smell-prone zones. Pine makes a powerful inhalation for treating respiratory infections, and when rubbed on the chest, it acts as an expectorant. Diluted and used on open wounds, pine will disinfect the area and speed the healing process.

Common name: Pine (Scotch)
Botanical name: Pinus sylvestris
Essence from: Dry needles, twigs, and cones
Cultivated in: Russia, Scandinavia, North America
Aroma: Sharp, fresh, forest
Perfume note: Middle

Common name: Rosemary
Botanical name:
Rosmarinus officianalis
Essence from: Flowers,
leaves, and twigs of herb
Cultivated in: East Africa,
Italy, Middle East,
France, Spain,
Aroma: Strong, fresh,
woody, herbaceous
Perfume note: Middle

In the West rosemary has a long and involved history. It has been honored and considered sacred in many ancient traditions. In Latin *Rosmarinus* means "Dew of the Sea," which refers to its preference for warm, sea-sprayed environments. Greek philosophers wore garlands of rosemary to stimulate the mind and promote memory. In wedding bouquets it is a symbol of fidelity, and in funeral rites as a remembrance of the dear departed. In the seventeenth century, the famous herbalist Nicholas Culpeper claimed it helped jaundice and failing eyesight, and healed open wounds. Charlemagne declared the herb should be grown in all his imperial gardens. Rosemary has been used to ward off evil spirits and was burned in sickrooms and hospitals to protect against epidemics. In the fourteenth century, Queen Elizabeth of Hungary used rosemary in facial water and rejuvenating cosmetics. It was supposed to have transformed a paralytic, gout-ridden old princess into a beautiful maiden who was wooed by the King of Poland. Rosemary transforms a dull skin to a translucent, radiant complexion and dry, lackluster hair into luxurious locks. *Benefits:* Rosemary is a great transformer. It brings inspiration to the dull mind, relief to the ailing, blood to the heart, and desire to the impotent. Rosemary is a nerve stimulant, energizing and activating the brain. Rosemary returns memory and helps improve eyesight and smell blindness. Mental strains, headaches, and vertigo can be helped by rosemary as can cardiac conditions and rheumatic pain. It is an effective antiseptic, antispasmodic, analgesic, and astringent, useful in treating many skin conditions such as dandruff, acne, and lice. *Safe use:* Applied to burns and wounds, rosemary speeds the healing process. When inhaled, rosemary stimulates the mind and brings balance to the nerves. In small doses in massage blends, this oil can help boost the circulation but it must be diluted (2–3 drops) for the bath. *Caution:* It's important to note that in small doses rosemary is stimulating and in large doses it's sedating. Rosemary should be avoided by epileptics and during pregnancy.

80

Common name: Sage
Botanical name: Salvia officinalis
Essence from: Leaves and flowers
Cultivated in: All over the world
Aroma: Herbaceous,
rich, heady, strong
Perfume note: Top

The Romans called sage *herba sacra*, or "sacred herb." Sage was the most celebrated of all medieval medicinal herbs, and was used to cure a multitude of ills—from migraines to foolishness. Sage is associated with eternal youth, probably because its essence contains sclareol, which is now used in perfumes because its scent mimics ambergris, an aphrodisiac. *Benefits:* This common, everyday garden herb hides its light under a bushel. Long hailed as a sacred herb, sage is a masterful healer, an antispasmodic, antiseptic, and general body tonic. It has been used to treat sluggish digestion, asthma, low blood pressure, and nervous afflictions of all kinds for centuries. As a mouthwash or gargle, sage has been known to treat ulcers, inflammations, and gum disease. Sage contains an estrogen-like substance that regulates menstrual flow. *Safe use:* In burners and infusions, sage will clear the atmosphere and relieve any nervous tension. Massaged into the skin in minute amounts, it will help digestion, asthma, fevers, menopause, reduce night sweats, stimulate the appetite, and treat skin infections. *Caution:* Like rosemary, sage is stimulating in small doses and sedating in large doses. Sage can be toxic if it is overused and should be avoided during pregnancy and nursing.

Common name: Rose Otto
Botanical name: Rosa centifolia/
Rosa damascena (Damask Rose)
Essence from: Flowers
Cultivated in: Morocco, Turkey, Bulgaria
Aroma: Deep floral, rich, sweet
Perfume note: Middle

Fossil specimens indicate that some varieties of rose have been growing in North America for more than thirty-two million years. The adaptable rose has been cultivated and crossed for many centuries. The rose is featured on the walls of Egyptian and Abyssinian tombs dating back to 500 B.C. The great Cleopatra used the luscious flowers in her cosmetics and bathed in the petals regularly. King Midas's rose garden was one of the wonders of the ancient world. The Romans are largely responsible for the widespread use of rose. They planted herb and rose gardens everywhere they conquered. In Greek and Roman mythology, the rose is linked to the goddess of love, Aphrodite and Venus. The rose color is said to be the bloodstains Aphrodite left when she pricked her fingers on the thorns. Other stories report that Cupid spilled wine on the shrub or that he shot an arrow into the heart of the bush. The rose is the ultimate token of love and like love, it stimulates the senses—it's intoxicating. Medieval herbalists recorded the healing properties of the rose and waxed lyrical about its agreeable, sweet, feminine aroma. The rose has been compared to women for centuries—its open, sensual, soft shape and enticing aroma embody the essence of woman. Legend has it that rose oil was first discovered during a wedding feast in Persia. The canal surrounding the royal palace was filled with roses and as the sun's heat beat across the surface of the water, the oil separated and floated to the top. The oil was collected and the merchant-minded Persians made a killing. Today the best and most expensive oil comes from Bulgaria, where it's extracted from damask roses. It takes approximately thirty roses to make a single drop of the precious oil. *Benefits:* The "Queen of Flowers," rose is the court physician. Rose ministers well to women—it is an emmenagogue, which means that it has an effect on the hormones, regulating menstruation and relieving the symptoms of PMS. Rose has been known to cure sterility and is the preferred aphrodisiac of queens and princesses, courtiers and commoners alike. Rose is an impressive liver and spleen tonic, it stimulates bile secretion, and purifies the blood. Rose is a splendid antidepressant and it is said that those who smell the sweet aroma are addicted for life. It strengthens the heart and tones the skin and capillaries. Rose is said to balance the yin and yang, or male and female energies of both men and women. *Safe use:* Rose is the least toxic of all the essential oils. It is useful for almost every skin type and is helpful for treating the dryness associated with mature skin. Infused into the atmosphere or dropped into a bath, it brings feelings of bliss and contentment. It can be a useful treatment for postpartum depression.

Of all the aromatics, sandalwood has the strongest tradition of use in Eastern religious rites. In China and India, sandalwood has taken on the same significance that frankincense has in Western religious ceremonies. In China, sandalwood is known as *chan-t'an*, derived from the Indian Sanskrit *chandana*. *Tan* means "true" and "sincere," and relates to the use of the wood as incense. As a part of funeral practices, sandalwood is often burned while the body is being cremated and then afterward as sign of respect for the deceased. Hindu holy men make a yellow paste and apply it to their foreheads as a symbol of their spirituality. The Indians have used sandalwood for more than a millennium to treat urinary problems. Chinese medicine has employed sandalwood to treat acne, nausea, and hiccups. *Benefits:* Sandalwood takes you on a heady journey to the garden of earthly delights. This versatile oil is exquisite in aromatic blends, baths, and burners, and an effective treatment for all skin types but especially dry, dehydrated skin. Massaged into the skin, sandalwood treats cystitis and urinary tract infections, laryngitis and autoimmune deficiencies and all persistent infections. Sandalwood has a powerful decongestant action and helps eliminate bacteria. This oil is a good cardiotonic, as it helps regulate the heart. Sandalwood is said to promote clarity of thought and induce deep meditative states as it sedates the nervous system. *Safe use:* Suitable for skin tonics, baths, infusions, and perfumes.

Common name: Sandalwood
Botanical name: Santalum album
Essence from: Wood
Cultivated in: India, Indonesia, Tonga, East Africa
Aroma: Soft, rich, sweet, woody, balsamic
Perfume note: Base

Common name: Tea Tree
Botanical name: Melaleuca alternifolia
Essence from: Leaves
Cultivated in: Australia
Aroma: Strong, medicinal, eucalyptuslike, refreshing
Perfume note: Middle

Having a sophisticated system of herbal medicine, the Australian Aborigines recognized the healing powers of tea tree many thousands of years ago, and used it to treat wounds and infections. Captain James Cook used the fragrant leaves in a substitute for tea, which is the origin of the name. The impressive antiseptic powers of tea tree were noted in the early 1930s and the leaves were used when medicines were in short supply. Tea tree was included in World War II first aid kits for servicemen posted to tropical areas as well as in ammunition factories where skin injuries were frequent. *Benefits:* The traveler's best friend, tea tree goes where angels fear to tread. This oil is a profound antiseptic and antiviral agent. Tea tree treats a multitude of ills—fungus, insect bites, itches of unknown origin, murky mucus, and various discharges. Tea tree is an effective treatment for chicken pox, shingles, cold sores, herpes, vaginal thrush, gangrene, candida, athlete's foot, ringworm, sunburn, hemorrhoids, and many of the recurring infections associated with chronic viruses. Unlike red thyme or oregano, which have potent antiseptic actions, tea tree is mild on the skin. A valiant warrior, it protects healthy tissue and defends damaged cells from attack by germs. Uplifting and stimulating, it is good for postshock victims. *Safe use:* Tea tree can be a bit rough when used undiluted on mucous membranes and open wounds, but many aromatherapists dab a minute amount right onto sores or acne. *Caution:* The best idea is to do a patch test before using tea tree on the skin, because it can burn (particularly people with sensitive skin). Not recommended for baths, as it can irritate sensitive areas. A couple of drops mixed with vodka and pure water can make an effective douche to treat thrush. As an inhalation, it is a powerful treatment for any respiratory tract infections or for treating conditions linked to low immunity.

83

In the Malay tongue, *ylang-ylang* or *Alan-ilang* means "flower of flowers." The tree is also known as the "crown of the East" or the "perfume tree." Ylang-ylang is one of the principal ingredients in Macassar oil, a nineteenth-century preparation used to encourage hair growth. In the Molucca Islands, ylang-ylang was mixed with coconut oil and rubbed over the entire body, warding off disease and leaving bodies in a fragrant veil. The Indonesians spread newlyweds' beds with the petals of the exotic flower to proffer luck, harmony, and fertility. Ylang-ylang is a famed aphrodisiac, which explains its wide use in perfumery. *Benefits:* Ylang-ylang is paradise found. It's a fragrant path that brings pleasure to the mind and body. Ylang-ylang is a great harmonizer, resolving internal conflicts, stimulating the emotions, and creating feelings of peace and warmth. The other trick ylang-ylang has up its sleeve is its ability to incite passion. For frigid lovers, ylang-ylang can ignite the essential spark. As a treatment for high blood pressure, depression, shock, and panic, ylang-ylang is a quiet river for the senses, regulating the flow of adrenaline and sedating the nervous system. Ylang-ylang is a valuable antiseptic and treats intestinal and vaginal infections. Ylang-ylang is also an effective skin treatment and balances both oily and dry skin conditions. *Safe use:* Ylang-ylang is sumptuous in fragrances and dropped into baths or massage potions. Infused into the air, ylang-ylang will disperse negativity. *Caution:* "Less is more" is a wise maxim when it comes to ylang-ylang. In this case, too much of a good thing can cause headaches and nausea.

Common name: Ylang-Ylang
Botanical name: Cananga odorata
Essence from: Flowers
Cultivated in: Comoro Islands, Indonesia, Madagascar, Philippines
Aroma: Powerful floral, sweet, heavy, full, exotic
Perfume note: Base

aroma

How to use essential oils and natural

Aromatherapy is the fastest growing alternative and cosmetic therapy today—turning up in a myriad of practices and treatments. Essential oils should be used in a synergy of touch, smell, and feeling to absorb their healing benefits.

therapies to achieve peace of mind

The aim of aromatherapy is to find pathways for the essential oils to get inside the body. Throughout history therapists have found innovative ways to have the oils sniffed, caressed, swallowed, and diffused into the body. Aromatherapy isn't easy to label because it isn't one great, big, natural healing discipline: Aromatherapy is any therapy that employs essential oils to heal. Most aromatherapists use essential oils combined with massage, literally rubbing the oils into the skin, but essential oils can also be used to boost the benefits of reflexology, acupuncture, hypnotherapy, and other healing disciplines. Aromatherapists will also use essential oils in burners, baths, perfumes, and infusions to treat their patients. Aromatherapy as we know it today is a complex and incredibly versatile healing modality. By exploring all the wondrous smells and actions of essential oils, you will discover which ones work for you. New doors to health and well-being will open through massage, reflexology, baths, infusions, and mixing your own fragrant blends. This chapter reveals some of the healing disciplines that, together with essential oils, will help bring health and happiness to your life.

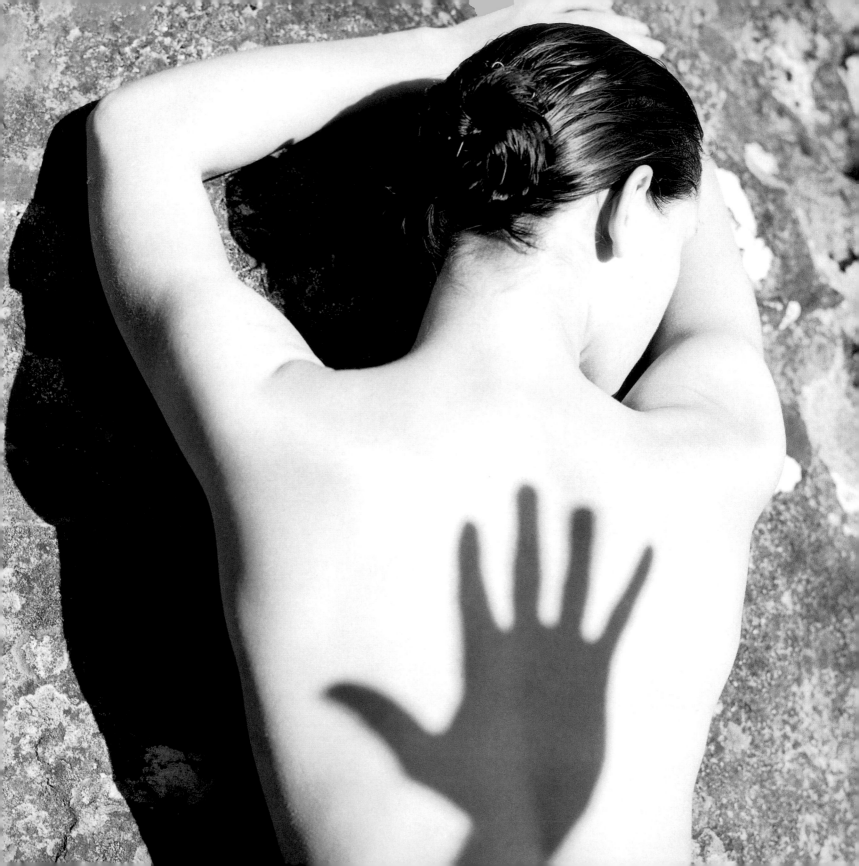

Massage

Sensual healing begins with the science of touch. Essential oils are enhanced by the power of a simple stroke—human contact. Learn to relax your mind, de-stress your body, and revive energy levels with these soothing therapies.

It's a natural human instinct to try to rub away pain. When you were young, your parents would rub a bruised knee, sore head, or aching stomach. Quite unconsciously we will massage our temples when we have a headache or pat our chest when we have indigestion. Recent research into pain behavior suggests that rubbing a sore spot will actually help the body's natural pain-blocking processes—touch receptors are stimulated that send nerve impulses to the brain, blocking its ability to register pain when the skin is rubbed. Skin translates all kinds of sensations from wet, dry, cold, and hot to pleasure and pain. Sensors in the skin are clever enough to distinguish between a feather tickling the skin and a needle prick, warning of danger or sending waves of delight to the brain and immune system. There are more touch receptors in the hands than in any other part of the body, which is the reason why massage is exciting for both the practitioner and the patient.

The skin is a complex organ that produces hormones and enzymes that are crucial to the immune system. Without touch, people become depressed and lackluster and can eventually wither and die. The skin needs many external stimuli to maintain proper health. It needs light, friction, good food, plenty of water, and lots of TLC. Massage can help soothe strains and pains, stress and emotional upset. It works like a dream on the cardiovascular system, the muscles, and lymphatic system. Massage can put an insomniac to sleep in minutes and conversely boost flagging energies in the lethargic.

The vascular system comprises blood and lymph, which flow throughout the body. Blood delivers fresh oxygen and lymph removes toxins, wastes, and bacteria that build up in the tissues. During massage, the movement of blood from the heart to the extremities and back again is speeded up—after a few minutes the oxygen content of the rubbed tissue has increased. The blood pressure drops during massage because the patient is relaxed, and the therapist's hands, not the heart, encourage the flow of blood and lymph; therefore, circulation is improved without exerting any energy. Most people's lymphatic systems are less than terrific. Lymph nodes in the armpits, neck, groin, chest, arms, and knees are supposed to filter all the body's wastes and purify them by adding anti-bodies and antitoxins. Sedentary lifestyles, stress, and unhealthy diets block the flow of lymph and can contribute to poor immunity, general malaise, and low-grade infections. Aromatherapy massage is generally designed to liberate lymph and speed the elimination of toxins from the body. Stress and irregular exercise also contribute to tight and sore muscles. The anxieties and stress associated with modern living leave many of us with tense muscles.

Lactic acid builds up in strained muscles, which is the reason they often feel tender to touch. The more tension in the muscles, the more blocked and sore they will feel—massage draws the toxins from the muscles, soothes away stress, and stimulates blood flow back to those muscles.

The aromatherapy massage

Massage techniques vary from practitioner to practitioner. There's no mystery to massage, anyone can do it—and by using the basic techniques, you can create your own personal brand of healing.

The origins of massage are hard to trace. People have used touch for healing since the beginning of time. The Egyptians practiced a form of reflexology and Hippocrates mentions massage in his work. Many of the therapies we use today were developed in the East, namely Japan and China. Shiatsu, acupressure, and reflexology were brought from Asia by therapists who had studied these ancient therapeutic disciplines. Even Swedish massage is based on Eastern therapeutic techniques. It was developed during the nineteenth century by the Swedish gymnast-physiologist Per Henrik Ling who had traveled to China to learn many ancient Chinese healing methods. The therapy that eventually became known as Swedish massage incorporates his moves and strokes with Chinese techniques. India also has a strong tradition of massage—head massage with essential oils is part of daily life in India.

Eastern healing modalities often concentrate on unblocking stilled energies within the body. They believe that the *qi*, *chi*, or life force can become blocked by stress, emotional upset, and disease, which in the long term will create serious illness and death. Most Eastern therapies work to liberate the chi and bring well-being to the body and soul. Massage is one of the best ways to release energy flow in the body and bring balance and peace of mind. You don't have to visit a professional massage therapist to receive the healing benefits of massage. Self-massage can be just as stimulating or relaxing as massaging a partner or friend. You can use massage to soothe a baby, comfort a friend, delight a partner, or relax your own mind and body.

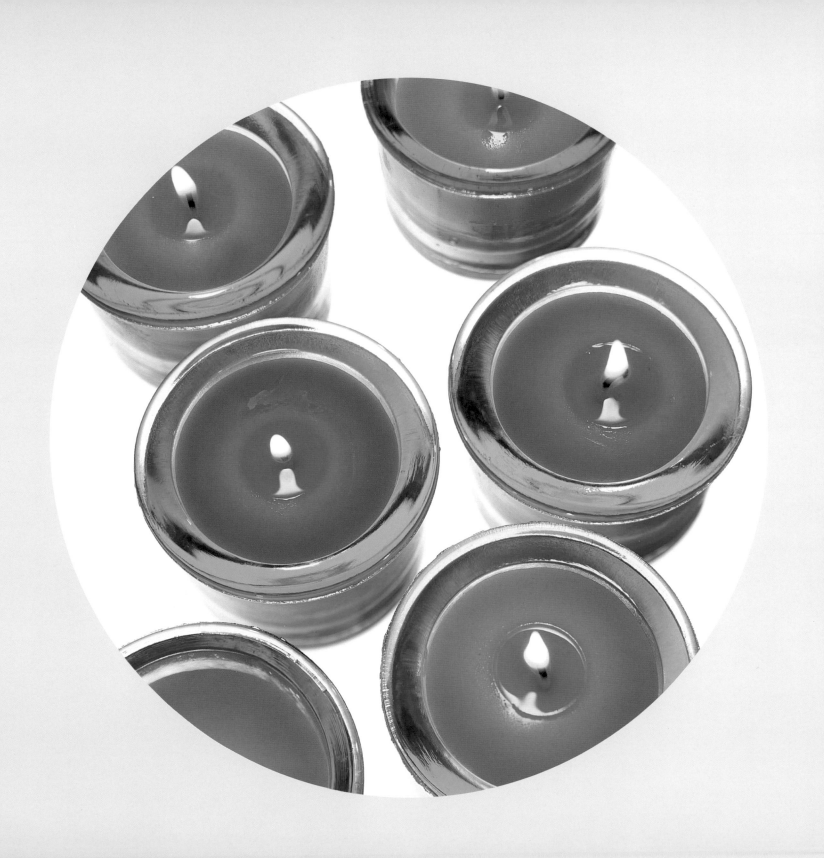

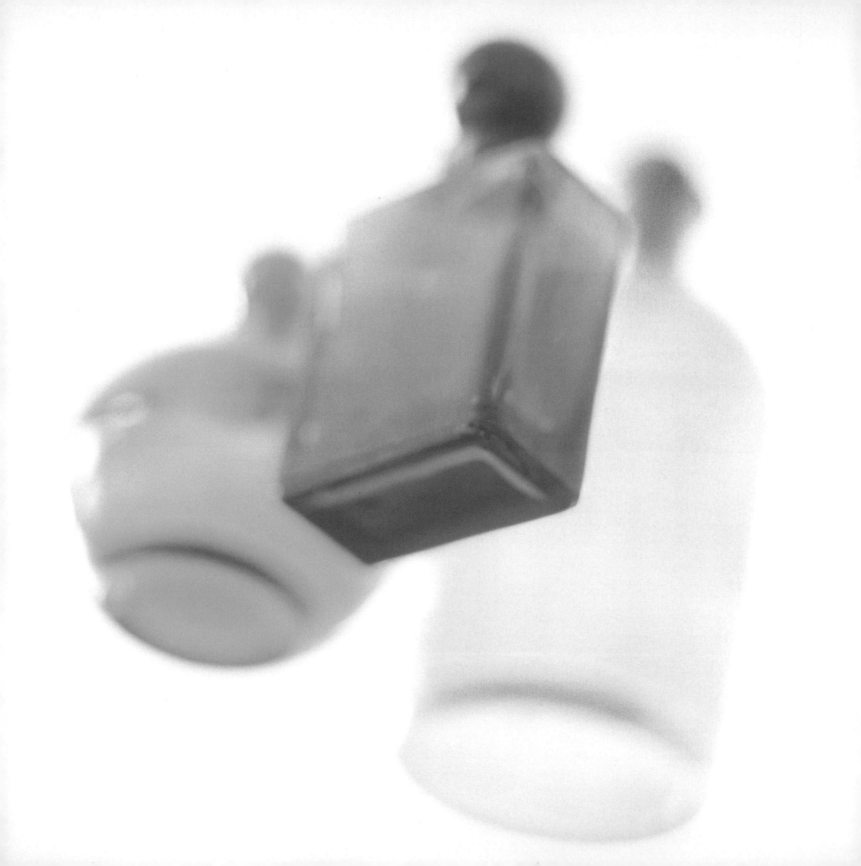

The beauty of aromatherapy is that you don't have to have a degree in biochemistry, a Ph.D. in psychology, or a master's in massage to apply the principles of this transformational art and science to yourself and your friends and family. However, because aromatherapy profoundly affects the body and emotions, there are a couple of things to keep in mind. Before any healing takes place, the practitioner must establish a relationship based on trust, care, and respect with the patient. Never treat beyond your knowledge and abilities—essential oils can be toxic in the wrong doses. Do not judge the experiences of the patient:

The art of aromatherapy lies in selecting the right essential oils and combining them with the best therapeutic practices. This is as much an intuitive as intellectual process. As a home-healer, or a lay-aromatherapist, you will find your greatest healing tool is your intuition. This nebulous sixth sense is in fact a primitive, instinctive faculty that keeps you in touch with your feelings and the feelings of others. The more you connect with your intuitive sense, the more acute and sensitive it will become. Many aromatherapists claim that by meditating or simply sitting in silence before prescribing an essential oil, or course of treatment, the right formula occurs quite naturally and easily.

Allow the patient to share his or her feelings with you. It is rare, but if you or your patient feels unwell after a treatment, or if a child swallows an essential oil, consult a physician immediately. It is always a good idea to consult a textbook to check on the dosage and toxicity of essential oils.

Start

If you do not have a professional massage table, you may find that the bed, couch, or even the kitchen table can be turned into a massage bench. Most professional masseurs work with a table because they can move around the body while they are massaging. It's important to be comfortable while you massage. For this reason, masseurs employ two main standing positions: the lunging position, which is mostly used to work over the large parts of the body, the back, legs, arms, and abdomen; and the squatting position, which is useful for working on the hands, feet, face, and head or areas that need a bit more attention. A good rule of thumb is to keep your back straight and your bottom tucked under and aligned with the hips. The lunging position involves standing with your legs a yard apart, one in front of the other, with the front knee facing the patient and the back leg straight behind you. To begin the squatting position, stand with the legs a yard apart. Point your toes outward and squat down, keeping your back straight. Each time you move from one area of the body to the next, remember to adjust your position to suit the stroke. You may want to sit while you work on the face and head or the hands and feet. Be careful not to strain your back while you work. Wash your hands before and after the massage and make sure you feel centered and calm before you begin.

The strokes

There are a number of touch techniques involved in massage. Remember that human touch reaches more than the superficial layer of the skin. Nurturing through touch is a powerful experience that can plumb the depths of the human spirit. Many people revel in the pleasure of nimble fingers working tension from muscles as they relax and unwind. However, those who have not been touched for a long time can experience deep emotions when they sink into the bliss of human contact. Long-stored emotions can bubble to the surface with a minimum of touch. Allow the patient, or yourself, to experience any emotion that may come up.

Effleurage

Effleurage consists of long, light stroking movements that prepare the skin for deeper touch. This stroke is usually employed at the beginning and end of a massage: It soothes the nervous system, warms the muscles, and stimulates the circulation of blood and lymph. Use both hands in successive strokes and glide them over the skin while applying an even pressure. The movements should be slow and gentle. Focus on bringing a calm state of mind to the patient and yourself.

Petrissage or kneading

This is a more energetic movement, performed in rhythmic rolling movements, lifting and squeezing the muscles with the hands. This helps encourage the flow of nutrients to the area and pumps away built up toxins and wastes, easing tension and tenderness. Use firm movements and take hold of the flesh between the thumb and fingers, pulling it away from the bone and kneading it like dough. This will promote blood flow and draw away stress. The shoulder and neck area will greatly benefit from this stroke.

Friction

This movement concentrates on one area of tension. Friction is usually carried out with the soft cushion of the thumb or fingers, though the strokes can be done with the heel of the hand on large areas. The part of the hand in contact with the area should knead in deep circular movements and slide over a path while circling. (It is advisable not to break contact with the body while massaging.) Friction will help break down fibrous knots and tension nodules, increasing the peripheral circulation.

Percussion or tapotement

Percussion is the slapping, cupping, and chopping movement used to stimulate or relax the nerves and break down fatty tissue. Depending on the length of time it is performed, it is said to improve muscle tone and firm slack skin. It is best used along the backs of the legs and the back. This movement needs to be performed in quick successive movements without breaking the rhythm.

Step-by-step one-hour massage

Back massage

Establish contact by stroking in upward movements, from the buttocks or base of the spine up to the shoulders and neck. Use the effleurage strokes in light, even movements to begin, and gradually increase the pressure. Use petrissage movements to warm up the muscles followed by friction. Although there is often not a great deal of flesh on the back, use kneading and squeezing movements on the shoulders, around the torso, hips, and buttocks. Use firm and even finger pressure to stimulate the spine, neck, and lower back, and run your two thumbs down the outside of the spine three or four times. Never press too hard and check what is comfortable for the patient. Use gentle percussion on the back and more energetic movements over the fatty areas of the hips and buttocks. Finish with long, careful effleurage strokes, as though you were stroking a pet, and work down the back and shoulders toward the bottom. This soothes and calms the nervous system and can bring the patient to a quiet state, close to sleep. *10–15 minutes*

Back leg and foot massage

Massage each leg individually. Start by stroking lightly down the leg, then up again to the buttocks, gently increasing the pressure with each stroke.

These stroking movements will stimulate the blood flow and boost lymph circulation. Use brisk friction movements on the back of the knee and ankle. Follow by working on the pressure points down the center of the leg and calf. Use petrissage and percussion movements on the fleshy parts of the thigh and calf, and then follow with effleurage movements, stroking slowly up and down the leg and circling the ankle with the thumbs. After completing the leg, rub the soles of the feet with even pressure. Press the heel of the hand into the arch of the foot, then rub the toes briskly between your fingers. Run the thumbs down the center of the foot using even pressure: This will stimulate the acupressure points in the foot, which have corresponding points in the rest of the body. When you have finished the feet, stroke slowly down the entire body with languorous, relaxing brushes. Now you can ask the person to roll over and begin on the front. *5 minutes per leg*

Arm massage

Massage each arm individually. Start by holding the patient's hand in your right or left hand (depending on whether you are right- or left-handed) and stroke gently down from the shoulder to the hand. Begin with the outer arm and work in toward the inside of the arm. Let the arm fall gently onto the table or bed and use petrissage to work your way up the arm, from hand to shoulder. Use both hands to knead the flesh and muscle of the upper arm, moving upward toward the shoulder. Use your thumb to apply pressure along the outer and inner arm, then stroke down the arm, and work over the hand. Repeat this movement several times to relax the muscles. You may want to use some cupping on the fleshy part of the upper arm. Massage the hand with the heel of your hand, pressing backward toward the wrist. Use firm, circular movements with your thumbs into the palm of the hand and massage the fingers by wriggling your fingers up and down the digits. Pull the fingers gently toward you and stroke the hands in rhythmic movements to finish. *5 minutes per arm*

Chest and stomach massage

Start with effleurage, stroking down from the neck over the décolletage and out toward the shoulders and armpits. Move your hands slowly over the neck and collarbone, stroking

down around the breasts and side of the torso. Gradually increase the pressure and work around the chest toward the waist. Some women do not like the nipples touched, so massage around the breasts in slow light motions. Knead and circle any sore points in the chest and upper abdomen, then use the palm of the hand to circle the stomach with firm clockwise strokes. Use petrissage to knead the flesh on the waist and hips, gently lifting the waist to drain any toxins away from the lower body. Stroke firmly and slowly from the rib cage, sliding the hands down in clockwise strokes over the stomach and repeat five to ten times. Finish by brushing the whole area gently and slowly with your fingers. *10 minutes*

Fronts of legs

Start by stroking the leg from the groin down to the foot. Use the same techniques you employed for the backs of the legs, kneading and cupping the fleshy parts of the front of the legs. Run your thumbs down the front and side of the thigh to stimulate the energy points. Massage the foot by running your fingers down the foot bones on the top of the foot and kneading the toes between your fingers.

To finish, sweep your hands over the entire length of the leg and gently squeeze the foot at the completion of each stroke.

5 minutes per leg

Head massage

Massaging the head can often be the most relaxing part of the massage, as it encourages the mind to become still and silent. Begin by lightly stroking the forehead and running the hands and fingers over the scalp and hair. Then, work in from the temples in small circular movements into the hair, and rub the whole scalp with the tips of your fingers, gradually increasing the pressure. After you have rubbed the scalp, move under the head to the back of the neck, and gently massage the head and neck with your fingers using small circular movements. Reach for the shoulders and press the tender points in the shoulders and upper back before you complete the massage. Stroke the head gently and brush your hands down over the forehead and crown to finish the massage, slowing the strokes as you go. Allow the person to rest for five minutes before you ask him or her to get up. Ask the patient to roll over onto his or her right side in the fetal position before rising. *10 minutes*

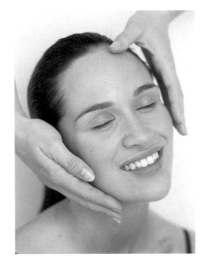

At the end of the session, when you have finished the last strokes, you may want to perform a simple cleansing exercise. Shake your arms and legs, as though you were shaking off a glove or a sock. After you have shaken your arms and legs five or so times, stand in silence with your eyes closed. Imagine a beautiful cooling waterfall cascading over your head and gently trickling down your body. Continue until you feel calm and relaxed. This technique will help you separate your energy from your patient's energy. During massage a special bond is made between the masseur or masseuse and the patient. It is often appropriate to reestablish your own space after the massage.

Mood

Massage is an intimate and private practice. When the massage is injected with the healing energy of care and trust, amazing physiological, emotional, and spiritual transformations can occur. Perhaps the most ancient form of healing is the laying on of hands—the deep communication of love and healing. Massage can make the patient feel nurtured and loved or exposed and vulnerable, having shed the clothes and emotional armor worn in daily life. Essential oils come into their own in massage because the healing aromas help lull the client into a peaceful state. If aromatherapy burners are lit before a patient enters the room, the atmosphere will be infused with lovely smells and the mood will be intimate and conducive to healing. Candlelight and soft music will also contribute to an atmosphere of trust, comfort, repose, and healing.

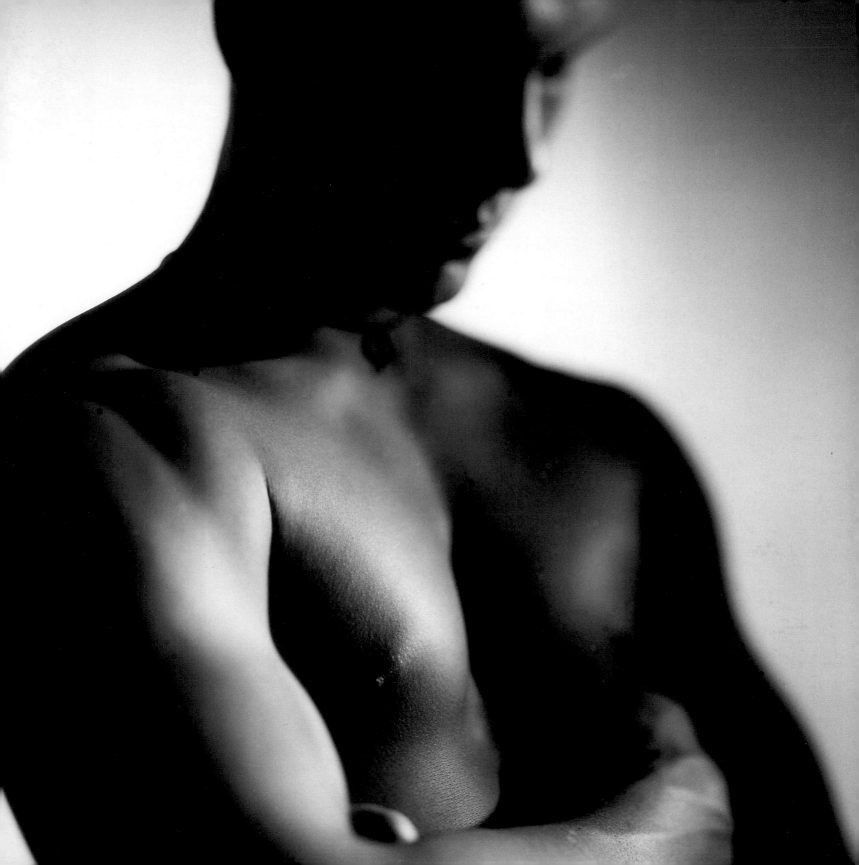

When not to massage

Generally, common sense will tell you when massage should be avoided, but you should consult a doctor or certified holistic therapist before you massage people with the following conditions:

1. an infection, a high temperature, a fever, or a contagious disease
2. recent surgery, broken bones, or an open wound or swelling
3. a skin eruption, such as severe acne, a chronic skin disease, eczema, or a rash
4. a heart condition, severe varicose veins, or other chronic circulatory problems
5. a history of back problems or acute back pain
6. the first day of menstruation
7. recent inoculations.

Wait two hours after a heavy meal before beginning a massage.

Massage is a great treatment for systemic infections like bronchitis and flu but some localized infections, such as boils, may be spread. Back pain may be relieved by some gentle rubbing or stroking, but only qualified practitioners should exert pressure on weak or sore backs. Under these conditions, a hand or foot massage may be safe and appropriate.

Massage and pregnancy

A gentle, loving touch during pregnancy is often welcomed by expecting mothers. It not only soothes the mother, but can sedate active babies intent on doing aerobics in the womb. Some essential oils are not suitable for pregnant women. These oils are listed in Chapter 5. Please check the actions of oils before prescribing or treating a pregnant woman with massage and essential oils. Again, check with a doctor or qualified practitioner before you begin. Focus on the legs, arms, head, feet, and back, as these areas are easier and safer to massage than the abdomen and chest. A pregnant woman may be more comfortable resting among a pile of cushions or on the bed, propped with pillows. The practitioner will need to ask the patient how she is feeling during the practice, as she may need to move and adjust herself.

During labor, massage and aromatherapy may be a positive and nurturing way for a partner to participate in the birth. Back and shoulder ache can be relieved with gentle rubbing and pressing, but do not use any pressure strokes on the abdomen or anywhere on the torso. Massaging the feet can also relieve tension and bring comfort to the woman in labor. It is important to rest between contractions, so a face massage, softly pressing on points around the eyes, temples, and mouth, can be very relaxing.

There is probably no better time to gently massage and pamper a woman than after childbirth. The body is exhausted, and a loving touch from a friend or partner may be the world's best medicine. Keep the movements soft and flowing and do not take any strokes to a level of discomfort.

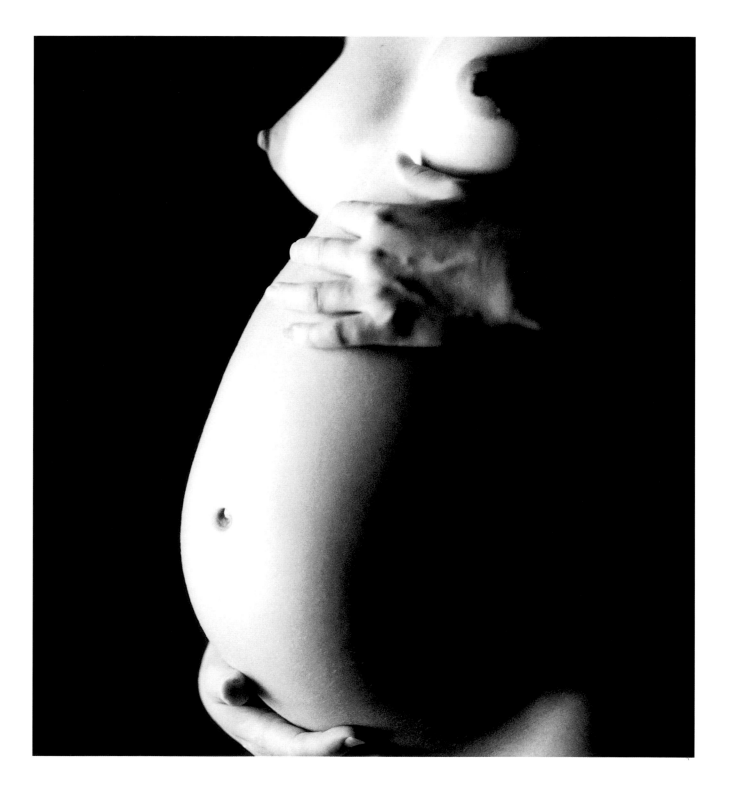

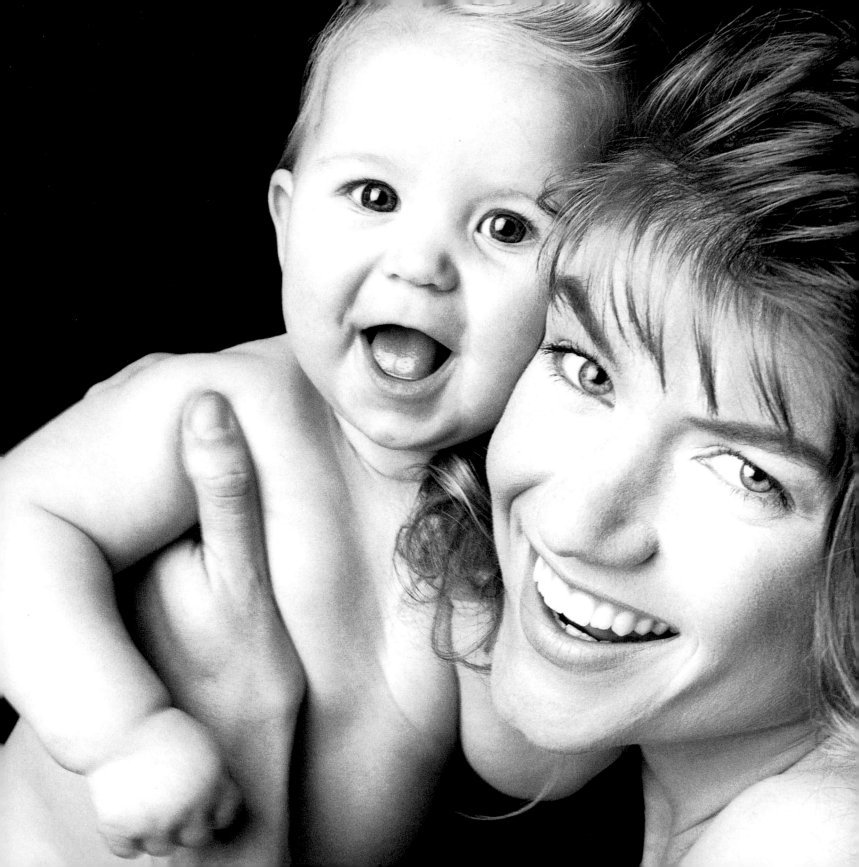

Baby massage

Babies cannot survive without touch. In India, a mother will massage her baby from birth and will continue to touch her family in a nurturing and therapeutic way while they live with her. Baby massage works in much the same way as animals licking their young. Licking serves to stimulate the physiological systems and aid the bonding process. Massage in human babies speeds the development of the nervous system and the brain.

Aromatherapy massage can help balance all the baby's developing systems and encourage optimum growth.

Remember: Babies can be bruised and hurt. Any massage should be done with extreme care and stopped immediately if the baby reacts badly.

Aromatherapy massage for infants should be done with a light, but firm hand and a special aromatic baby oil, which is best made yourself with good quality vegetable oils. Many commercially available baby oils are made with mineral oils, which can dry the skin. A baby formula should never contain more than 2 drops of essential oil per 1³/4 fl oz of carrier oil. Lavender, rose, and chamomile are the generally accepted essential oils for babies and will often prevent cradle cap and diaper rash. Massage will generally delight children, particularly restless and

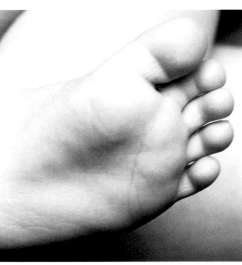

colicky babies. The experience will stay with the child as a blissful memory and massaged infants are often calm, focused, and quick to learn. The smell of lavender or rose will activate a flood of pleasurable memories of being touched and cared for.

Legs and feet

Babies reach out to the world with their legs and feet. Babies also "defend" their torso from the outside world with their legs and feet, the least vulnerable parts of their bodies. For these reasons, baby massage begins with the feet.

Start with the Indian Milking technique, which involves squeezing down the inside leg with both hands—one following the other. The outside hand is used to stabilize the body as it's squeezing down the leg and the other hand immediately follows. Massage each leg individually, and repeat strokes five times. The next step involves taking the foot and pressing along the sole with your thumbs in firm but shallow movements. Then, take the foot in one hand and squeeze each toe gently. Next, take the ankle and run your thumbs around the ankle and press gently into the tops of the feet with your thumbs. Finish the legs with the Rolling technique, which involves gently rolling the leg between both hands from ankle to knee in much the same way as you would roll dough between your palms.

The stomach and chest

This stroke for the stomach will tone the baby's intestinal system and help relieve any gas or constipation. Begin by stroking from the rib cage down, using clockwise motions in small, shallow circles. The next move is the Water Wheel, which is a paddling stroke that involves moving one hand after the other, gently scooping the baby's tummy toward the feet—like scooping sand toward you. Follow by kneading the baby's tummy gently with the flats of your thumbs, working from the center of the stomach out toward the sides. The next stroke begins in the center of the chest, sweeping both hands toward either side of the rib cage. Then perform the Butterfly stroke, a diagonal movement from one shoulder across the chest to the bottom of the rib cage. This stroke should be performed rhythmically, crisscrossing the chest, alternating from left to right.

Arms and hands

The arms should be treated in the same way as the legs. With the baby still on its back, take the arms and extend them out toward you, "milking" the muscles by squeezing and rolling the flesh as your hand descends down the arm from the hands. Stroke the armpit gently with small circular movements. Then, open the baby's hand with your thumbs and roll each finger between your index finger and thumb. Stroke the top of the hand and the palm. Then massage the wrist, making small circles all around.

The face

Babies can become quite tense and often hold a lot of stress in their faces. Sucking, teething, crying, and eating can make the muscles tight and sore. Using the flats of your fingers, start in the middle of the forehead and push out toward the temples. With the thumbs, press lightly over the eyes, then sweep down over the bridge of the nose and across the cheeks. Next, sweep your thumbs across the upper lip and slide the fingers under the chin and up to the jaw bone where you can make small circles with your fingertips. To finish, gently glide your hands over the forehead and down the back of the head.

The back

Back massage can often be the most relaxing part of the baby massage and can put little ones to sleep. Turn the baby onto its tummy with its legs outstretched and arms by its sides. Start by moving your hands back and forth over the back from the shoulders and neck down to the buttocks and up again. Then, keeping its bottom stationary, sweep one hand up from the buttocks toward the neck. Make small circles all around the back with your fingertips. Then spread your fingers apart and run the index finger and middle finger gently down the outside of the spine from the neck down to the buttocks. Repeat five times. Finally, sweep your fingers down from the head to the buttocks in gentle, soothing strokes.

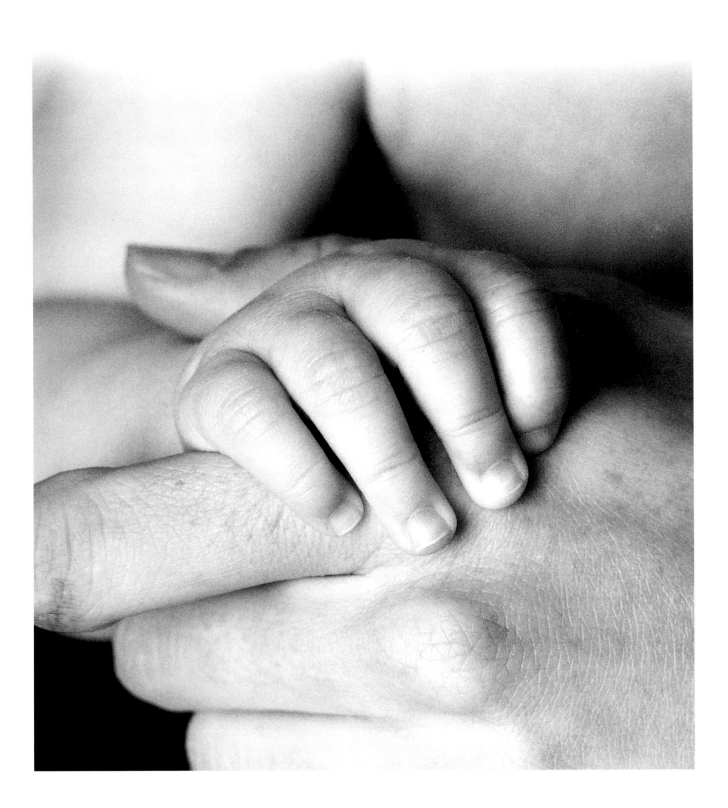

Reflexology Chart

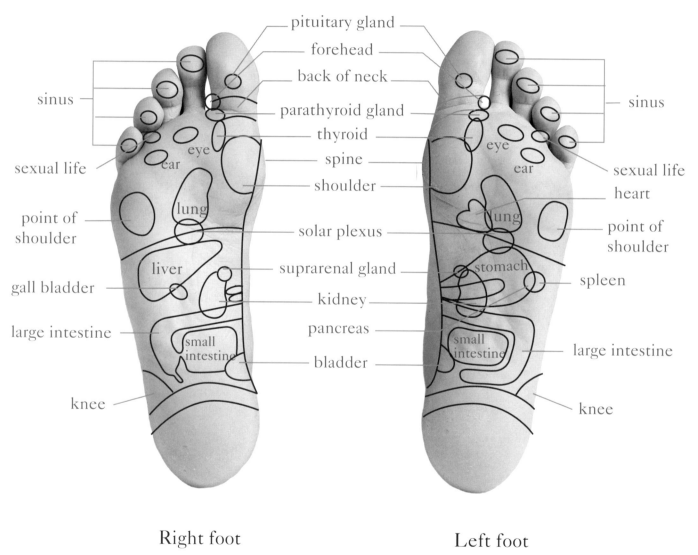

pituitary gland

forehead

back of neck

parathyroid gland

thyroid

spine

shoulder

solar plexus

suprarenal gland

kidney

pancreas

bladder

sinus

sexual life

point of
shoulder

gall bladder

large intestine

knee

eye

ear

lung

liver

small
intestine

sinus

sexual life

heart

point of
shoulder

spleen

large intestine

knee

eye

ear

lung

stomach

small
intestine

Right foot

Left foot

The healing art of reflexology

Reflexology is an ancient practice that dates as far back as Egyptian times. Since then, many other indigenous medical systems have used pressure points located on the hands and feet to heal. Modern reflexology has its roots in the early twentieth century, when Dr. William Fitzgerald, an American physician, suggested there were specific interactions between zones on the hands and feet and the major organs. He believed that pressure on particular points on the feet and hands could send messages along energy pathways and reach the organs. In reflexology, the body is divided into zones, or energy channels, five on either side of the body's midline, which runs from the top of the head to the feet. Any part of the body can be stimulated by working on the reflex area of the feet. For example, by pressing the inner arch of the foot, it is possible to activate the kidneys. This means that the hands and feet can be used to communicate healing energy to the internal organs.

Reflexologists believe poor diet, stress, lack of exercise, and illness can cause congestion in the feet, resulting in deposits of crystallinelike lumps around the nerve endings. By using deep pressure with the fingers, therapists can break down the structures (thought to be composed of waste materials). When the deposits are broken down by pressure and massage, they are eliminated from the body through the bloodstream. Reflexologists also use the therapy as a diagnostic tool. Tender areas in the foot can indicate congestion in other parts of the body. The therapist can feel the crunchy deposits and determine where in the body there is a blockage of energy.

There's no question that a foot massage can instantly relax and invigorate the body. Reflexologists recommend a daily foot massage to maintain good health. Regular attention to the feet will help ensure that toxins do not build up and the feet remain flexible and soft. During the 1930s Eunice Ingham, a physiotherapist and masseuse, developed a chart of reflex points that correspond to the rest of the body. By using the thumb and forefinger you can diagnose potential health problems. Although a qualified reflexologist will offer more specific advice, reflexology is a terrific diagnostic and healing tool that anyone can use.

Feet treat

Warm the foot with a relaxing foot bath that
includes a couple of drops of lavender, rosemary, or
peppermint essential oil. Gently dry the foot, stroking
with even pressure using both hands. Then, work over the
entire foot with the thumb in small, circular movements, or
repeatedly pressing and then releasing points to stimulate
the reflex. Use the reflex chart, referring to the organ zones
while you press tender spots. Essential oils can be used
effectively with reflexology. Therapists will often use
reflexology to make a diagnosis, then select an oil that will
benefit the points and corresponding organs. For example, the
aromatherapist or reflexologist may discover some crystalline structures in
the kidney area under the arch of the foot, and on closer examination, find the
patient gets urinary tract infections regularly. The therapist may recommend
further investigation by a doctor, but in the meantime may prescribe a few
drops of cedarwood and eucalyptus, which help flush the kidneys and
prevent congestion. Most people find a few tender spots on their
feet. They are generally not very serious, although you will
find that after working on the feet, over a period of
time the soreness will subside and eventually
disappear. This often corresponds with
an increase in energy and
enthusiasm.

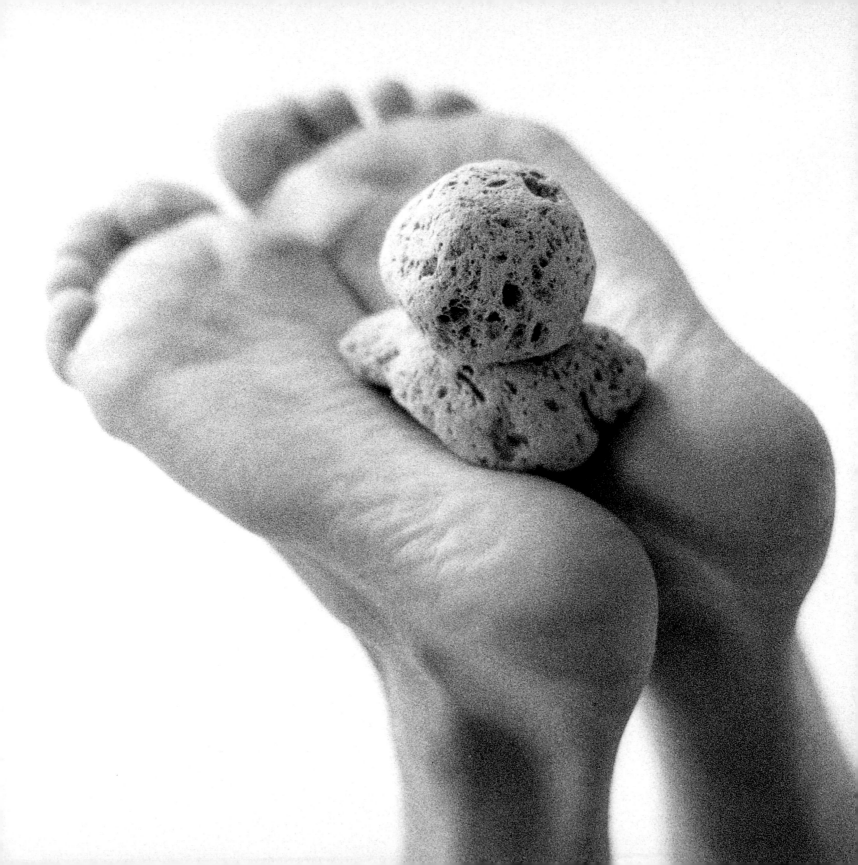

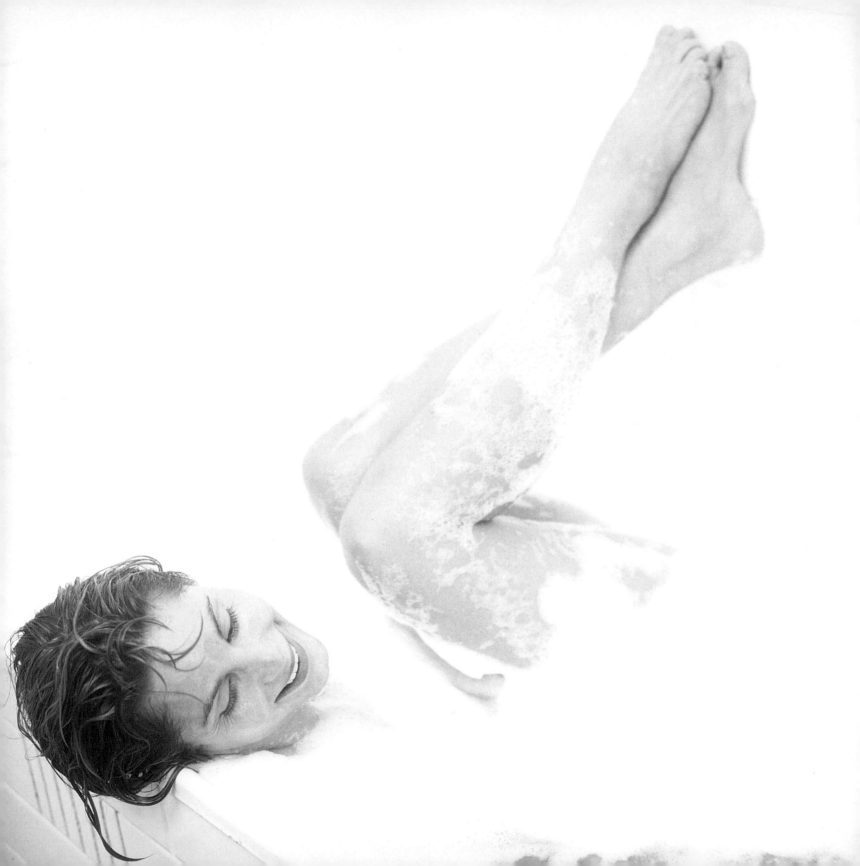

Bathing

The simplest biological forms began life in the Earth's primordial waters more than 3.5 billion years ago. As if to remind us of our watery origins, nature filled all living creatures with her own life-giving essence—water. All living creatures consist of two-thirds water. Without water life is not possible. Water is so essential to life that humans can live for many weeks without eating, but can survive a mere three to four days without water. Much of what appears to be the solid mass of the human body is actually water.

The fetus is gestated in a salty, mineralized bath that cushions it in the womb—we emerge from these protective waters into the dry, harsh world. Perhaps these are the reasons why bathing is one of our most instinctive impulses. Human beings have always worshiped water as the very source of life and have included bathing in religious rites and personal ritual. Mythology is filled with water gods and nymphs and all manner of sprites who live in the waters of the world.

Bathing has also long been associated with pleasure. Primitive plumbing has been found in Egypt, India, and Greece, but none rivaled the Romans for their balneal excitement.

The Roman bathing ritual was the first to combine elements of the aromatherapy bath. After entering the *thermae*, or bath room, the bather was rubbed down with essential oils and then encouraged to work up a sweat. The next step was to retreat to a sauna or steam room where a servant would exfoliate the skin with a blunt metal instrument. Then, the Roman sybarite would be cleansed with warm water, massaged, and left to soak in a warm bath. This was followed by a quick dip in an icy pool, which would stimulate the metabolism and speed the elimination of toxins from the body. This routine would often take up to five hours, and was completed with a last stop at the *Unctuarium*, where rare and wonderful perfumes were applied to the body in a rigorous rubdown.

Few of us have time to indulge in five-hour bathing rituals, but aromatherapy baths are a wonderful way to treat the skin, relax the muscles, and bring the mind to a quiet state. Water softens the skin and allows essential oils to penetrate the dermis.

Skin brushing

The actions of essential oils work best on clean skin, free from dry, dead surface cells. Dry brushing with a loofah or a natural bristle brush is a terrific way to prepare the skin for an aromatherapy bath or massage. Dry brushing is a form of self-massage that is widely practiced in many Scandinavian countries. It stimulates the circulation and aids the elimination of toxins from the body while it sheds dead skin cells.

Rub 1 drop of a mild essential oil, like rose or lavender, onto the brush to sterilize it, and start by brushing your feet. First the soles, toes, and tops of the feet and ankle, then work your way up the leg toward the thigh. The buttocks and upper thigh will benefit from regular gentle brushing—the skin will glow and the microcirculation will improve. Brush up the arms, paying special attention to the elbows and forearms. Finally, work up over the abdomen and torso in small circular movements. This action will stimulate the colon and help break up the fatty deposits on the stomach. Leave the breasts and nipples out of the routine, and concentrate on the upper chest and shoulders. Be careful to avoid any moles on your back that you can't see.

Aromatherapy baths

The bath is a tranquil haven in an otherwise frantic world. The trickling water, steam, and heat banish anxieties and provide space in which to unwind and rejuvenate. The Japanese and Koreans still view bathing as an art rather than a necessity; they rinse and wash the body clean before they even step into the bath. In order to gain the full benefits of an aromatherapy bath, you must allow sufficient time to relax and enjoy its simple pleasures.

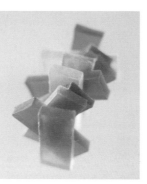

The temperature of the water will often dictate how much time you spend in the bath. Warm water will provide the best environment for you to luxuriate, and will allow anything from a five-minute cleanse to an hour soak. Very hot water will make the heart beat faster and can be dangerous for people with infections, fevers, and heart conditions, and the elderly. As alcohol dilates the blood vessels, it is not advisable to enter a hot bath intoxicated. Cold baths are said to benefit the circulation and regulate the heart, and in some northern European countries, Korea, and Japan, cold baths are used for religious and therapeutic purposes.

However, cold baths are unlikely to relax an overtaxed nervous system or nurture tired bodies after a long day in the concrete jungle. An aromatherapy bath in warm water will do the trick.

Adding essential oils to your bath will enhance your pleasure and boost the oils' effectiveness. They soak easily into the skin and are inhaled with every breath, soothing the muscles and mind simultaneously. The steam carries more aroma molecules to your nose than when you burn them in burners or wear them as fragrances. This means that the smell is more potent, pleasurable, and powerful. The best way to use essential oils in the bath is to drop them in drop by drop after you have turned the taps off. The oils will float on the surface of the water and will coat your skin as you lower yourself into the tub. The molecules of oil will hover in the air for more than fifteen minutes, but your nose will stop registering the scent after a few minutes as it tires of the stimulation. Don't be tempted to pour more oils into the bath. The oils will continue to work long after your sense of smell stops detecting them. When it comes to essential oil baths, less is often more. Essential oils can have quite contradictory actions; for example, peppermint can be a powerful digestive, but in high doses can cause nausea. Although it is safe to drop many oils undiluted into the bath, you can reduce the risk of sensitivity by mixing them with a nourishing carrier oil that will also treat the skin. Six to 8 drops for adults, and 2 to 3 drops mixed

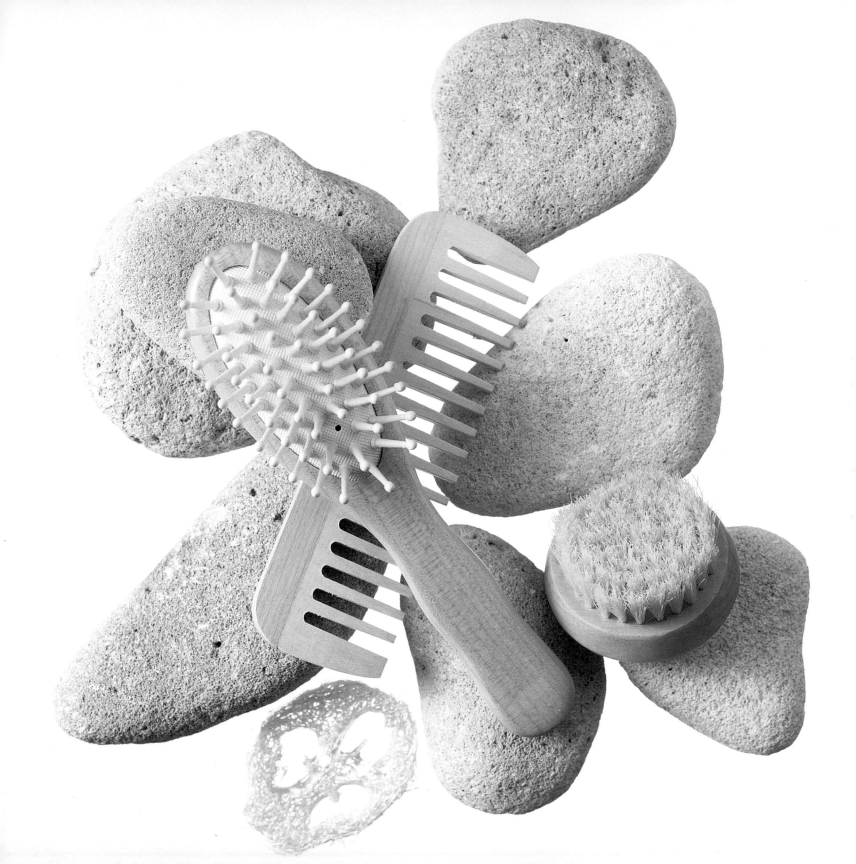

with vegetable oil for children, are generally safe for a single bath; however, some very potent oils require far fewer. The therapeutic benefits are the same as when you apply essential oils in massage, but you may find that, because more molecules are available to the nose, some oils will be more acceptable than others to your olfactory palate. You will find that if you are turned off by an essential oil in the bottle, that experience will be magnified in the bath. Use your intuition as well as your sense of smell to determine which oils to drop into your bath.

A comprehensive guide to blends and recipes is included in Chapter 5 of this book. Use it to determine the aromatic powers of different essential oils. For example, don't pour relaxing oils into the bath if you have an important appointment that demands your complete attention, and be aware that stimulating oils dropped into a bath before bedtime may keep you up. The heat of the bath will increase the oil's ability to penetrate, so be careful not to go overboard. Check the lists included in Chapter 5 for information on which oils are suitable for bathing.

Burning and infusion

The Latin word *spiritus* has two translations: It can mean "breath" or it can mean "inspiration from the gods." All living cells need the invisible gas oxygen to survive, which is the reason many religions assert that breathing is our connection to the divine, invisible spirit of the universe. While normal breathing accomplishes the elimination of one-third of the toxins produced by the body, inhaling essential oils is a good way to promote internal health, because they help stimulate the digestive process, respiration, and the nervous system.

Essential oils have been used in burners and baths for centuries. In sacred rituals, aromatic plants have been burned to clear the atmosphere of evil spirits and have been strategically placed on the body to protect the wearer from both physical and spiritual ills.

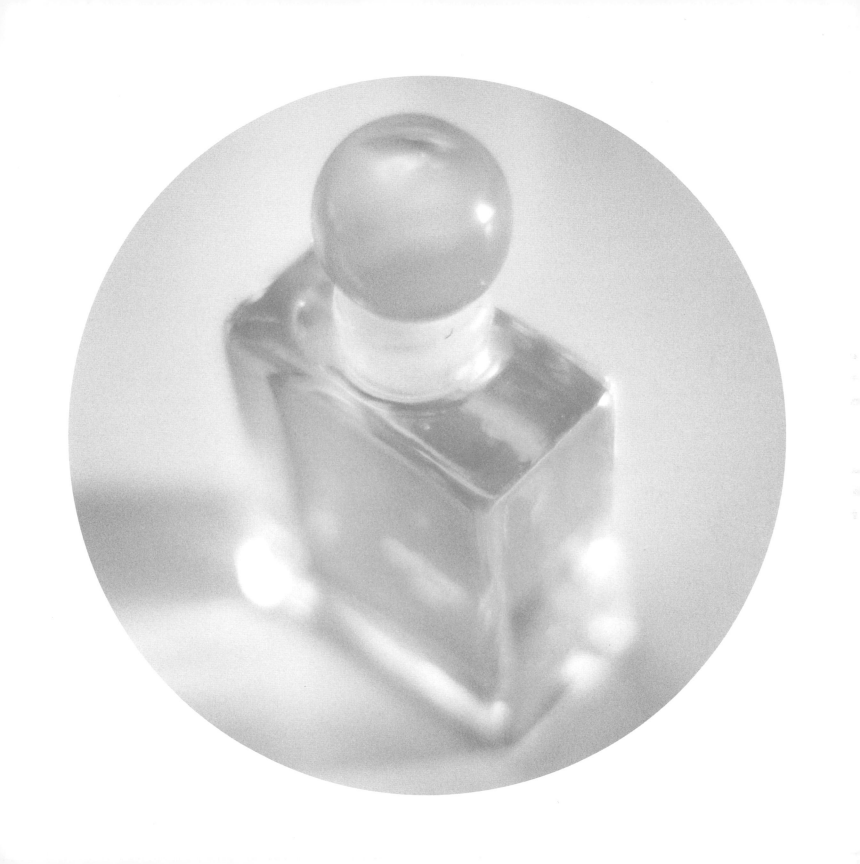

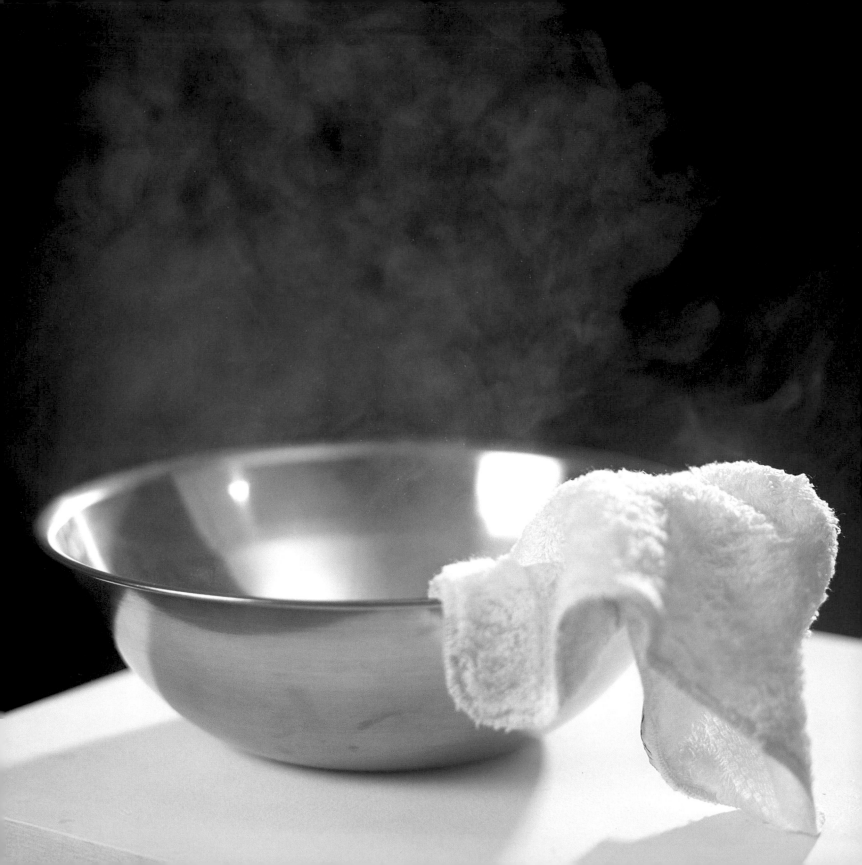

Essential oils are volatile, which means they become airborne as soon as they make contact with the atmosphere. Steam is a great essential oil carrier and can be used to disinfect the air in any enclosed environment. The vapors of lemon essential oil are said to neutralize the meningitis virus in fifteen minutes and the typhus bacillus in less than an hour. Many people use burners or vaporizers every day to keep their spirits high and the atmosphere free of airborne germs and bacteria. Essential oils have profound mood-enhancing abilities. You can alter the chemistry of the brain by using specific oil combinations. Therefore, it is possible to sedate or uplift people who smell the airborne molecules of oil. Electric or battery-operated vaporizers are extremely effective and can be the safest option for the nursery, but the low-tech burners that use a candle flame under a ceramic or metal bowl often work very well in any environment.

Essential oils dropped into a basin of hot water and breathed in will treat persistent coughs and colds in next to no time. This old-fashioned remedy works on the respiratory system and helps the body expel mucus, kills bacteria, and boosts immunity. Tea tree oil, eucalyptus, and pine are all effective against upper respiratory tract infections. It's a good idea to put a towel over the head while inhaling so the aromas are concentrated toward the nose. Keep the eyes closed to protect them from the powerful vapors. Eight to 10 drops will usually be sufficient.

Compresses

Applying an essential oil compress to relieve pain and swelling or a bite or wound is a fast and effective way to speed recovery. Arthritic joints, and menstrual and stomach pains, headaches, sprains, varicose veins, and sore muscles all benefit from this easy and efficient treatment. Compresses can be cold or hot depending on the type of injury or pain. Hot compresses are most often used to treat pain of a chronic nature and cold compresses to treat acute pain, as a first aid for injuries such as sprains. Insect bites are usually treated with a cold compress because heat can spread the poison, and menstrual or arthritis pain are better treated with a warm compress. There are many schools of thought as to whether sprains should be treated with hot or cold compresses, but usually a cold compress is called for (check with a physician if in doubt). Use a natural fiber cloth (cotton is best), and pour 2 or 3 drops of essential oil into the water and disperse with your fingers. Wring the water out of the cloth and apply it directly to the sore spot. Wrapping the area with plastic wrap or an old sock can help keep the compress in place. Generally, compresses should be left on the affected area for at least fifteen minutes; however, warm compresses will chill quickly and may need to be replaced frequently.

- Hot compresses are particularly helpful in the treatment of backache, menstrual pain, rheumatic and arthritic pain, earache, and toothache.
- Cold compresses are helpful for headaches, sprains, tennis elbow, and other inflamed or swollen conditions.
- Hot compresses dilate, or open, the blood vessels, bringing more blood to the area. Cold compresses constrict, or shrink, the blood supply.

By alternating hot and cold you can create a flushing effect, helping drain excess fluid and toxins from the area. This technique may be useful in the treatment of sprains or sore muscles after a rigorous workout. Always start with a hot compress and finish with a cold one.

Caution: Do not apply compresses to large areas of the body of children or the elderly.

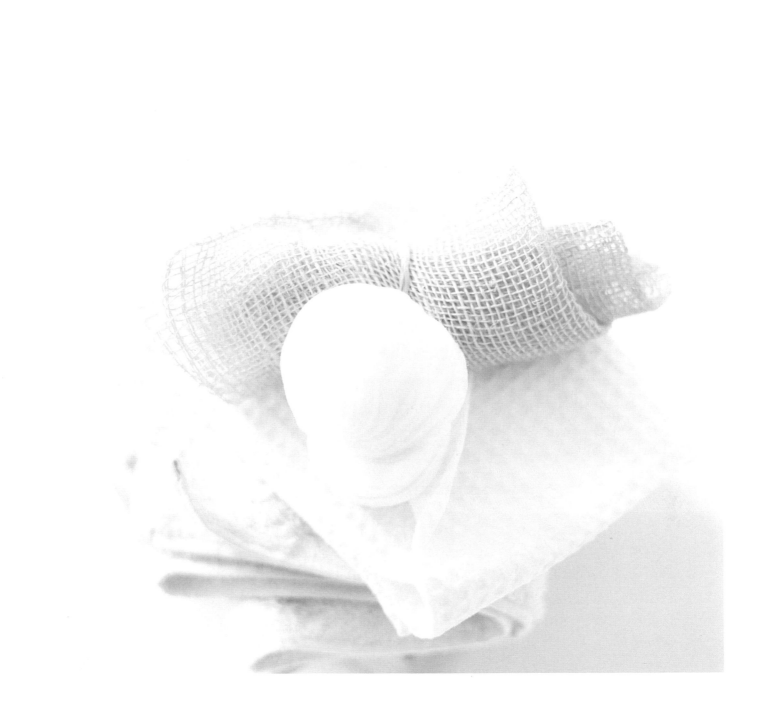

The aromatherapy facial

Cleopatra was probably the first, or at least the most famous, cosmetic aesthetician. She knew how to harness the powers of aromatic plants to heal and treat the skin. Performing her daily cleansing in rose baths, and using scented creams and ointments on her face, she became versed in the science of beauty therapy. Essential oils have an incredible affinity with the skin's own molecular processes as well as possessing anti-aging properties, which make them terrific cosmetic treatment aids.

Modern aromatherapy is being embraced by the cosmetic industry as the demand for plant-based products grows. A facial is often a fast track to relaxation as well as an effective treatment for your skin. Essential oils can help anything from oily and acne-prone skin to dry and sensitive skin conditions. (Recipes for skin treatments are included in Chapter 5.)

The following step-by-step aromatherapy facial has been adapted from aromatherapist David Wehner.

1. Cleanse the face and remove all makeup. David suggests a multipurpose liquid soap or olive oil and glycerine, which can be used over the whole body. Milk on a moist cotton ball can also cleanse the skin and remove makeup.

2. Make a compress by dropping 2 or 3 drops of pure lemon or lavender oil in very hot water and immersing a small towel into the water. Wring excess water and, while still steaming, gently wrap the face in the towel, patting it down over the face. This simple hydration process performed regularly (ideally every morning) will help balance the skin, reduce the formation of blackheads, and refine the pores. Men will find this treatment will soften the beard and make shaving easier. This process will also aid people with breathing problems or colds and flu.

3. Remove the towel when cooling and pat the face dry with a clean cloth.

4. Spritz the face with a gentle astringent such as witch hazel or a floral water made from distilled water with lavender, rose, and neroli essential oil added.

5. Apply a gentle scrub to the face, neck, and décolletage. Mix 1 tablespoon of ground almonds together with a teaspoon of natural honey (a powerful antiseptic and healing agent). Apply in gentle circular movements. Allow to dry for 10–20 minutes, then rinse off with warm lavender water.

6. Apply a mask made from powdered green clay. Clay powder is available from many health food stores and can be mixed with witch hazel, water, and essential oils. A drop of peppermint oil will help clear blemishes and revitalize dull complexions, and a drop of lavender will soothe and calm sensitive or irritated skin. Alternatively, mixing a drop of a mild oil such as chamomile, rose or geranium to the mask will boost any skin type.

7. Finish the regimen by moisturizing the skin. Dampen the skin with warm water before

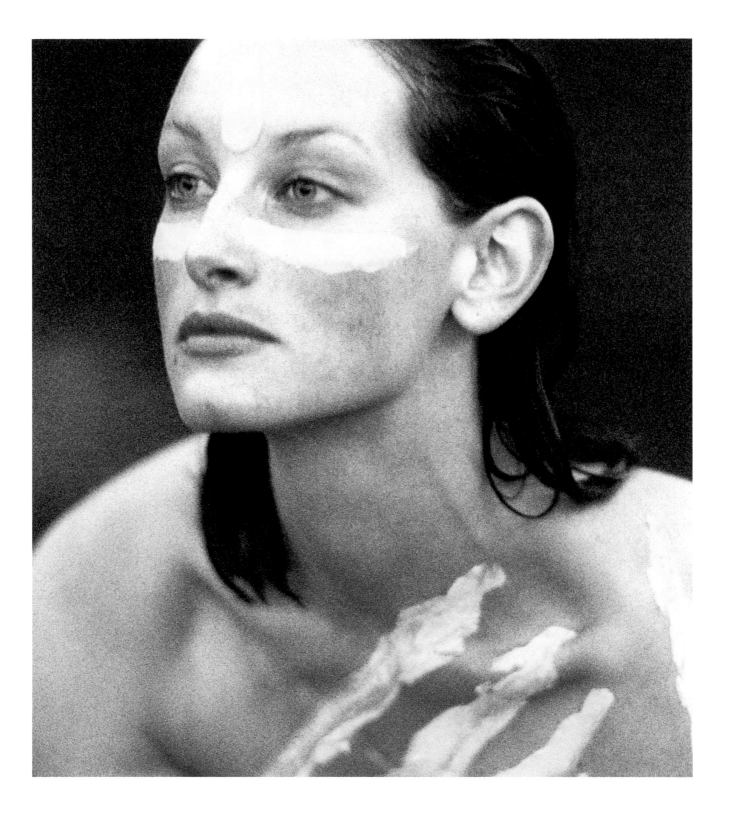

applying the moisturizer. Blend carrot oil with equal amounts of evening primrose and vitamin E oil. If you like, add a couple of drops of rose, lavender, or neroli to this formula.

The reason aromatherapy has become so popular in recent times is that people need feel-good therapies in their lives. Simply put, individuals are searching for solutions to the stresses of modern life—treatments that make them feel positive, uplifted, revived, and happy. Disillusioned with conventional healing methods, men

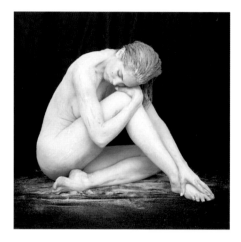

and women, young and old, are turning to alternative practices to provide simple strategies to treat the mind, body, and spirit. Under the right conditions, essential oils can act as powerful catalysts for health, and when combined in a synergy of touch, smell, and feeling, their benefits can be magnified. Aromatherapy is a profoundly sensual practice. It awakens the senses and stimulates all systems of the body. Being touched and enveloped in heavenly scent can give you a feeling of being nurtured, soothed, bathed in pleasure, and cared for. And the miracle of aromatherapy is that it works instantly, anywhere, and at any time. A burner on a desk at work is a simple way to bring well-being to everyone in the office; a few drops of lavender worn as a perfume will help bring balance to the mind all day long; a couple of drops of peppermint oil in a footbath at the end of the day will help you relax and unwind, washing away the stresses of the day. It's amazing how much healing can come from these little practices.

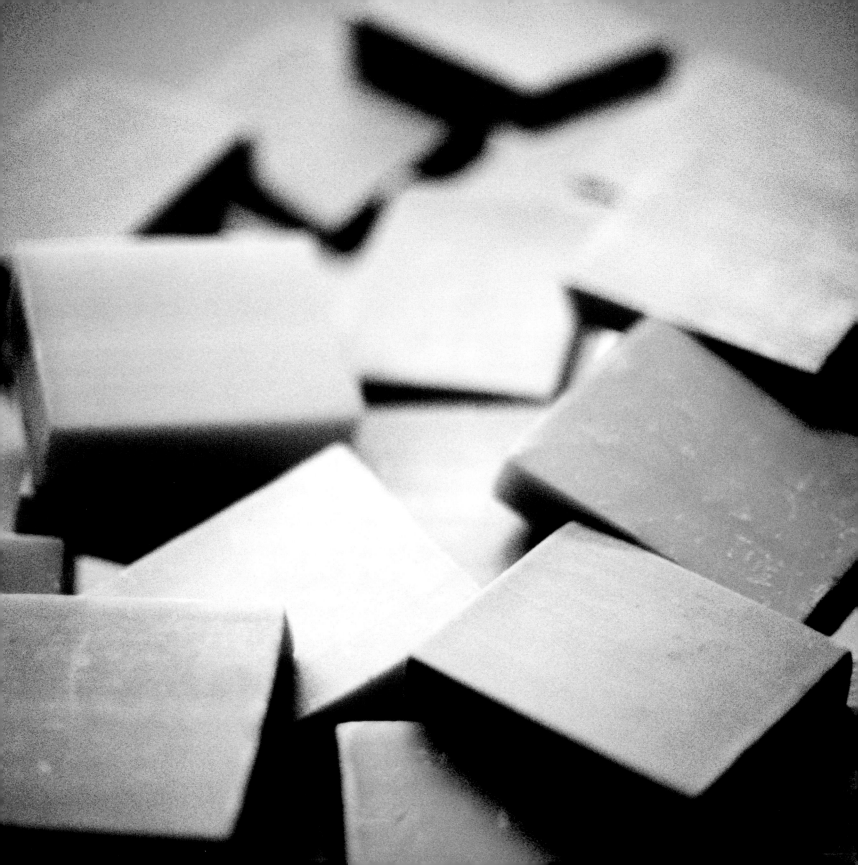

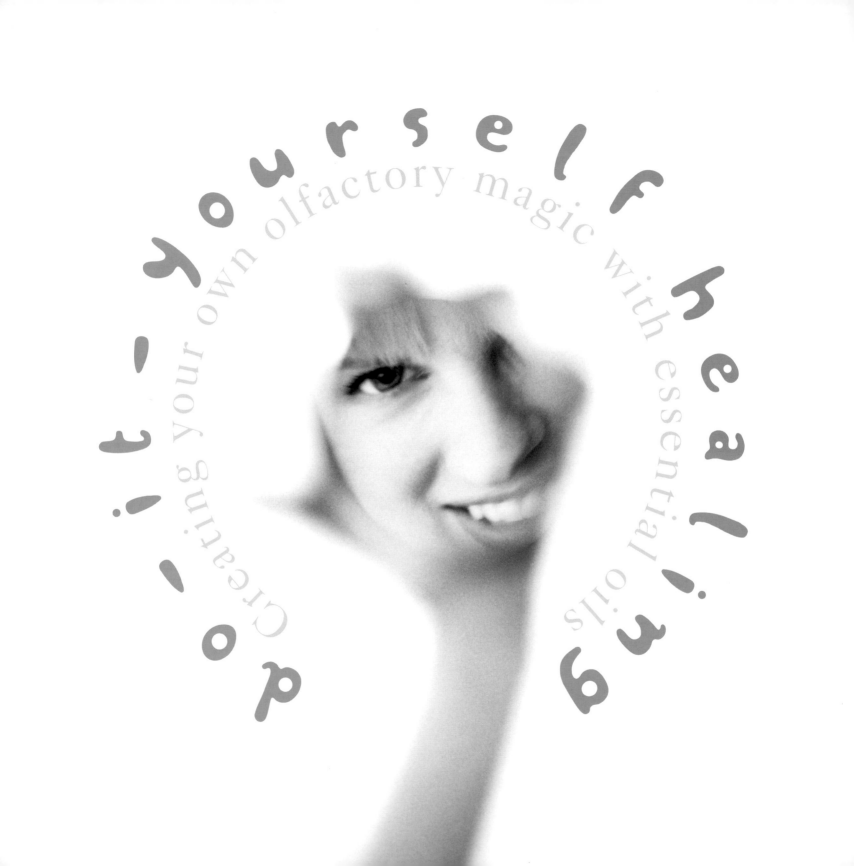

do-it-yourself healing

Creating your own olfactory magic with essential oils

Aromatherapy
opens up a fragrant
paradise for the body and mind,
a place where the stresses of the world
dissolve into nothingness. Like the alchemists of
old, you can mix your own potions and perfumes,
uncovering a pathway to a new realm of sensual healing.
When essential oils are blended they become the most
amazing medicinal perfumes. Although fine fragrances are often
designed to have an impact on the emotions and the senses,
essential oil perfumes and blends differ in one important way—they
are made from pure ingredients and there are no synthetic chemicals
in the formulas. Many fine perfumes contain essential oils, but only
in low concentrations. Some perfumers would argue that even the
tiniest molecules of essential oil can have a profound effect on the
mind and body, but for the purposes of aromatherapy,
unadulterated essences are preferable for their health-
giving benefits. Blending essential oils is an important
part of aromatherapy. On their own, essential oils
can smell inviting and sumptuous or sometimes
slightly offensive, but when they come together,
the harmonious combinations of
scents are nothing short of
magnificent.

Essential oils can be classified as top, middle, and base notes. The concept actually comes from the fragrance industry, which developed aroma notes as an easy way of determining an oil's staying power. Top notes are essential oils or compounds that are the most volatile, meaning they evaporate quickly. Middle notes are less volatile and the base notes are those that evaporate slowly. The top note is the aroma you smell first and it generally evaporates as the fragrance "dries down," or sinks into the skin. The middle notes linger and are often known as the heart of the fragrance, providing the body of the scent. The base note is generally the smell you detect last and is often included in a fragrance to fix the odor and enable it to linger.

The language of perfume is borrowed from the language of music. Anyone who has been moved by the power of music will also know the pleasures of scent. The single odors are known as notes and the blends are often called fragrant harmonies, light accords, and scentual symphonies. Fragrances have accents on particular notes, usually top notes, and the entire concoction has its own olfactory rhythm.

Some aromatherapists link the therapeutic effects of essential oils with the notes. Top notes are said to be the most stimulating and uplifting, middle notes can be stimulating as well as sedative, and are associated with the physical functions of the body, such as digestion and metabolism, and base notes are deemed to be the most sedating, relaxing, and grounding of all the oils.

Blending three oils—a top note, middle note, and a base note—will most often give you a harmonious blend. But there are no hard and fast rules. Let your nose and that of your patient guide you in your blending. You will know when a blend simply smells "wrong." It may not smell terrible, but you may "feel" it isn't a perfect combination. Your intuition is the most important source for discovering which oils will best treat a particular condition. Although textbook definitions will guide you through the time-tested therapeutic actions of oils, there is nothing like your own nose to determine what will work best at a particular time.

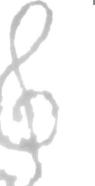

Top notes: basil, bergamot, chamomile, clary sage, eucalyptus, grapefruit, lemon, lemongrass, orange, peppermint, rosemary, sage, tea tree.

Middle notes: cinnamon, clove, fennel, geranium, juniper, lavender, melissa, petitgrain, pine, rose, tangerine, thyme.

Base notes: cedarwood, cinnamon, clove bud, frankincense, jasmine, marjoram, myrrh, neroli, patchouli, sandalwood, ylang-ylang.

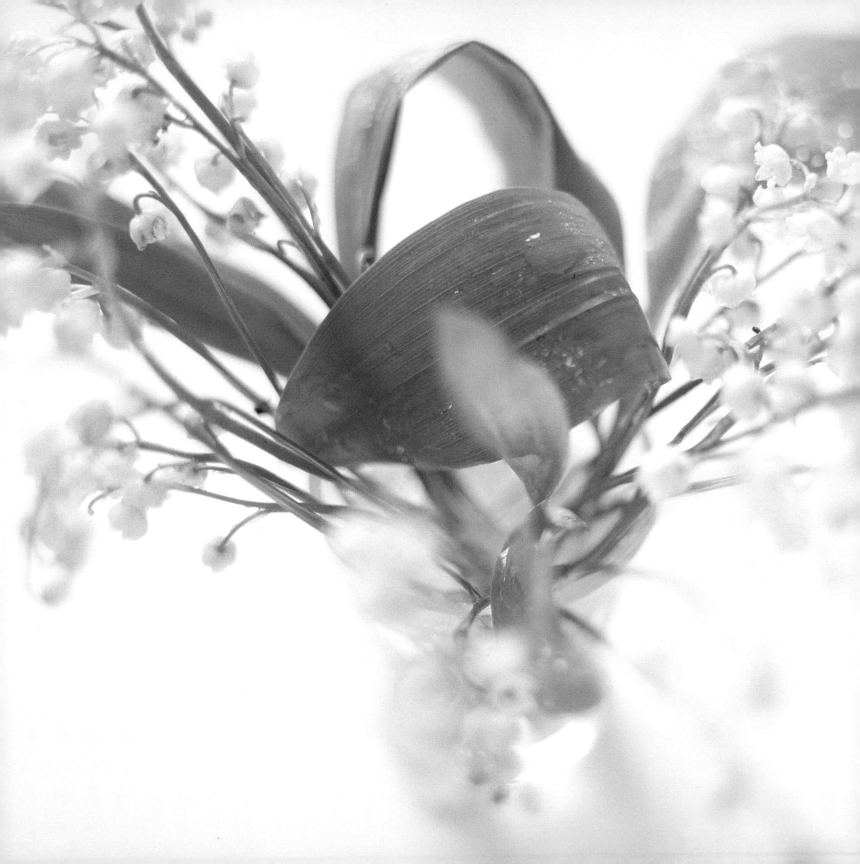

Perfumes

Creating your own perfumes can be inspiring,

sensual, and fun. You can perform olfactory magic by mixing

fragrant potions that uplift the mind, arouse prospective partners,

or boost low energies. There is nothing more enticing than an aura of

exotic and exciting scent. It will please everyone around you. Balmy summer

days may call for a light citrus scent while heady florals like jamine and ylang-

ylang may be perfect for a romantic dinner for two by the fireside. Mix your

fragrances according to your moods, lifestyle, or occasion and remember that

essential oil perfumes treat the body as well as the emotions. The strength of your

scent will depend on the ratio of essential oil to base oil, alcohol, or water. As

a general rule, perfumes use a dilution of 10 percent, eaux de toilette usually contain

about 5 percent dilution, and eaux de colognes, atomizers, and splashes mostly

employ a 1 percent dilution. Pure alcohol is often used for perfumes, but

if that does not appeal to you, jojoba oil makes an ideal base because it

does not turn rancid, and treats your skin while you wear the

scent. To create a refreshing cologne or spray, simply

add essential oils to distilled water and pour

them into an atomizer.

"The modern woman who dabs her body with expensive perfume
is attempting to acquire the irresistible sexuality of flowers."

—Tom Robbins, *Jitterbug Perfume*

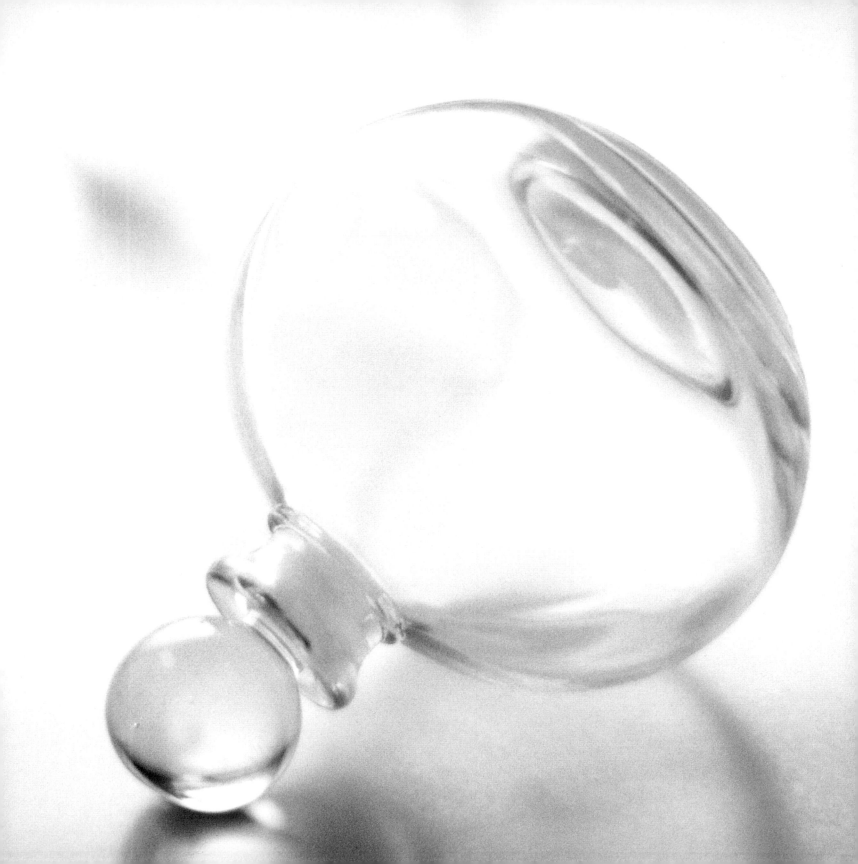

Blending Suggestions

Basil: bergamot, clary sage, geranium, grapefruit, jasmine, orange, peppermint, rosemary, sage.

Fennel: geranium, lavender, peppermint, rosemary, tea tree.

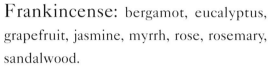

Bergamot: basil, cedarwood, chamomile, clary sage, frankincense, geranium, grapefruit, jasmine, juniper, lavender, lemongrass, neroli, patchouli, rose, sage, sandalwood, tea tree, ylang-ylang.

Frankincense: bergamot, eucalyptus, grapefruit, jasmine, myrrh, rose, rosemary, sandalwood.

Cedarwood: bergamot, clary sage, eucalyptus, geranium, jasmine, juniper, lavender, neroli, pine, rosemary, sandalwood.

Geranium: basil, bergamot, cedarwood, chamomile, clary sage, fennel, jasmine, juniper, lavender, lemongrass, neroli, orange, patchouli, rose, sandalwood.

Chamomile: bergamot, lavender.

Grapefruit: basil, bergamot, clary sage, eucalyptus, jasmine, juniper, lavender, lemongrass, neroli, rose, rosemary, sage, sandalwood, tea tree.

Cinnamon: bergamot, frankincense, grapefruit, lemon, orange.

Clary Sage: basil, bergamot, cedarwood, geranium, grapefruit, jasmine, juniper, lavender, pine, sandalwood, ylang-ylang.

Jasmine: basil, bergamot, cedarwood, clary sage, frankincense, geranium, grapefruit, lavender, neroli, rose, sandalwood, ylang-ylang.

Clove Bud: cinnamon, lavender, orange, patchouli.

Juniper: bergamot, cedarwood, clary sage, geranium, grapefruit, myrrh, pine, rose, sandalwood.

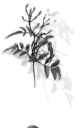

Eucalyptus: cedarwood, frankincense, grapefruit, peppermint, rosemary, sage, tea tree.

Lavender: bergamot, cedarwood, chamomile, clary sage, fennel, geranium, grapefruit, jasmine, lemon, myrrh, neroli, patchouli, rose, rosemary, sandalwood, tea tree, ylang-ylang.

Pine: cedarwood, clary sage, frankincense, juniper, lemongrass, marjoram, myrrh, neroli, orange, sage, sandalwood.

Lemon: lavender, neroli, orange, sage.

Rose Otto: bergamot, fennel, frankincense, geranium, grapefruit, jasmine, juniper, lavender, neroli, patchouli, sandalwood, ylang-ylang.

Lemongrass: bergamot, geranium, grapefruit, marjoram, neroli, pine, rosemary.

Marjoram: lemongrass, neroli, orange, rosemary, sandalwood, tea tree.

Rosemary: basil, bergamot, cedarwood, eucalyptus, fennel, frankincense, grapefruit, lavender, lemongrass, marjoram, peppermint, tea tree.

Myrrh: frankincense, juniper, lavender, patchouli, pine, sandalwood.

Neroli: bergamot, cedarwood, frankincense, geranium, jasmine, lavender, lemon, marjoram, myrrh, orange, patchouli, pine, rose, sage, sandalwood, ylang-ylang.

Sage: basil, bergamot, eucalyptus, grapefruit, lemon, neroli, orange, pine, tea tree.

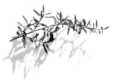

Sandalwood: bergamot, cedarwood, clary sage, fennel, frankincense, geranium, grapefruit, jasmine, juniper, lavender, marjoram, myrrh, neroli, rose, ylang-ylang.

Orange: basil, geranium, lemon, marjoram, neroli, patchouli, pine, sage.

Patchouli: bergamot, geranium, lavender, myrrh, neroli, orange, rose.

Tea tree: bergamot, pine, eucalyptus, frankincense, grapefruit, lavender, marjoram, myrrh, neroli, rosemary, sage.

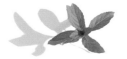

Peppermint: basil, eucalyptus, fennel, lavender, rosemary.

Ylang-ylang: bergamot, clary sage, jasmine, lavender, neroli, rose, sandalwood.

Carrier oils

Carriers are any substances that can "carry" essential oils into the body. Air is a carrier—the molecules of oil are transported to the nose through the atmosphere. Water is also a carrier. When essential oils are dropped into the bath they travel on steam through the air to the nose and penetrate the skin as the water washes over the body. All aromatherapy skin creams, lotions, shampoos, and body products are simply carriers that enable the essential oils contained in them to be absorbed into the body.

Carriers are most often cold-pressed vegetable oils, which act as natural and nutritious vehicles for essential oils. Carrier or base oils also dilute the essential oils.

The best carrier oils are fresh vegetable oils that have not been chemically treated. These oils are more perishable than supermarket oils and should be checked for rancidity. Once opened, they are best kept in the refrigerator.

Essential oils themselves will last between three and six years, although citrus oils will deteriorate more quickly (usually between twelve and eighteen months). Essential oils are also sensitive to sunlight, so individual oils and blends will stay fresher in either dark blue or brown bottles. Plastic can be degraded by essential oils—so store your blends in dark glass bottles away from sunlight.

Caution: If you see an essential oil being sold in a clear glass bottle, check with the retailer—it may not be a pure oil.

Mineral oils, petroleum jelly, and silicone oils are common ingredients in many commercially available cosmetics and skin care products. Mineral oils have an occlusive effect on the skin; that is, they form a barrier which prevents the evaporation of water through the skin, which can be beneficial in hot, humid climates where the skin can easily become dehydrated. But this occlusive effect can sometimes create fluid retention and cause irritations. Mineral oil and petroleum jelly have been shown to be allergenic in some cases and the substances can also cause the formation of blackheads and acne. Prolonged use of mineral oil can strip the skin of its own natural oils and cause it to become dry and flaky. Finally, mineral oil can also make the skin more photosensitive.

Recommended carrier oils

Sweet Almond: The aroma of sweet almond oil is mild and the oil is protein-rich and nourishing for the skin. It contains vitamins A, B_1, B_2, and B_6 as well as a small amount of vitamin E. Sweet almond oil is popular for massage and skin care because it has a long shelf life and will blend very well with other carrier oils.

Apricot Kernel: This oil is often more expensive than sweet almond oil, but it has similar actions. Often a key ingredient in facial tonics and cosmetics, this oil treats mature and sensitive skins successfully.

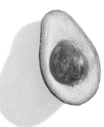

Avocado: A nourishing, rich, and heavy oil that is often blended with other cold-pressed oils for increased penetration. Avocado is often found in facial preparations because it is an effective treatment for dry and dehydrated skin. The unrefined oil is green in color and contains vitamins A, B_1, B_2, and E as well as lecithin. This oil also has a mild sunscreen.

Carrot: Carrot oil is rich in beta-carotene, vitamins B, C, D, and E, and essential fatty acids. This oil also has an anti-inflammatory action, which makes it a useful treatment for burns. Carrot is often used as an anti-aging treatment and is commonly found in skin creams. This oil can be too strong to be used on its own, but blended with olive and almond, carrot can be beneficial in facial blends.

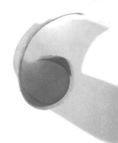

Coconut: Coconut oil is highly saturated, which means it will remain stable for a long time, making it a useful ingredient in cosmetic preparations.

Evening Primrose: A good oil for treating dry and mature skin.

Grapeseed: A clear, fine polyunsaturated oil with no particular odor. Good for body massage, as it is not sticky and leaves a satiny coating on the skin.

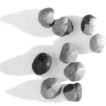

Hazelnut: Good for slightly oily skins, hazelnut is mildly astringent and will penetrate easily. This oil stimulates circulation, making it very good for muscular problems.

Jojoba: Although jojoba is a waxy liquid rather than an oil, it is often found in cosmetics because its powers of penetration are high and it does not become rancid. Excellent for hair and facial blends. (There is some evidence to suggest that jojoba may be an effective agent in the prevention of hair loss.)

Macadamia: This oil is high in palmitoleic acid, a monounsaturated fatty acid that is rarely found in vegetable oils, but is a natural component of skin sebum. It is an emollient oil and can be useful for the treatment of dry and mature skin.

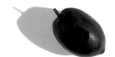

Olive: This oil will penetrate easily and soften the skin, but it has a strong aroma and is often best blended with other cold-pressed oils. Olive oil is warming and calming and is effective in the treatment of rheumatism and some skin disorders.

Rose Hip: Originating from Chile, harvested from a species of wild rose, this polyunsaturated oil has been used in clinical practice in topical applications with amazing results by Chilean dermatologists. Acne, eczema, seborrheic dermatitis, cracked skin, aged and sun-damaged skin, scars, stretch marks, burns, wounds, and overpigmented skin have all been shown to benefit from rose hip oil.

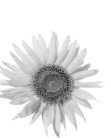

Sunflower: Good for all skin types, it has only a mild aroma. Sunflower oil contains vitamins A, B, D, E, and F, a source of unsaturated fatty acids that help control the metabolic rate and balance cholesterol levels. Vitamin F plays a role in the proper functioning of the skin and can help regulate sebaceous glands. This oil is good for treating skin conditions and dandruff as well as leg ulcers and bruises.

Wheatgerm: This heavy, rich oil is often too greasy to be used on its own, but when blended with other carrier oils it will help slow rancidity. The oil contains high concentrations of natural vitamin E.

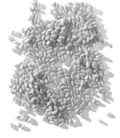

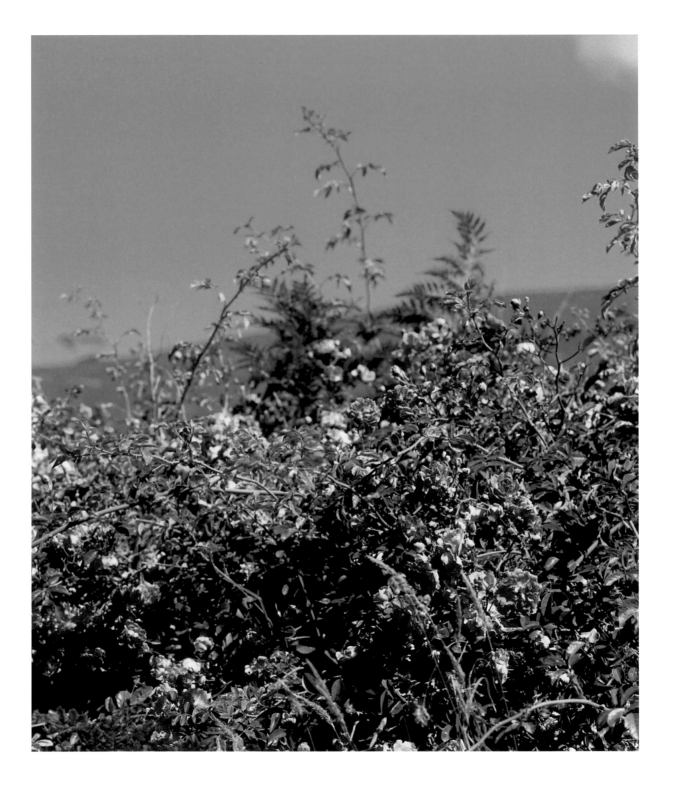

Carrier blends

Vegetable oil molecules are much larger than essential oil molecules, which means they are generally unable to pass through the skin and enter the blood stream. However, this does not mean that they are not benefical to the skin and useful in the treatment of some conditions. Carrier oils represent more than 95 percent of any massage mix and should be taken into account when treating skin conditions. These blends are a starting point. You can combine carrier oils as well as essential oils to create powerful healing blends.

The ratios

The ratio of essential oil to carrier oil should be between 8 and 12 drops of essential oil for every $\frac{1}{2}$ fl oz of carrier oil for baths or massage mixes. For facial blends, most aromatherapists will use around 6–8 drops to every $\frac{1}{2}$ fl oz. Mild oils like lavender and rose have been known to be blended in higher concentrations of 12 drops to every $\frac{1}{2}$ fl oz, but 10 drops are usually safe. The size of the drop of oil will depend on the device used. The thickness and viscosity of individual oils will also change the size of the drops dispensed. Lateral droppers, which are generally inserted into the mouth of the bottle, will give larger drops than pipettes or eyedroppers. If your essential oil bottle does not come with a dropper, most pharmacies sell eyedroppers. Again, err on the side of caution and drop only small quantities of essential oils into your blends—or perform a patch test on the forearm, waiting 15–20 minutes before applying the blend to the face or body.

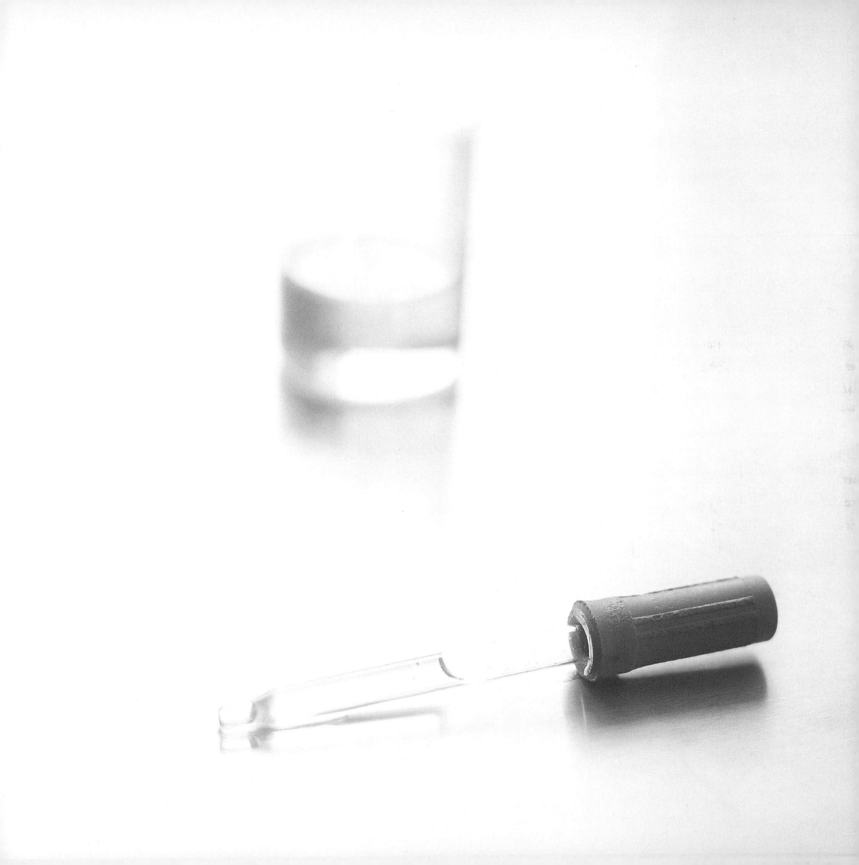

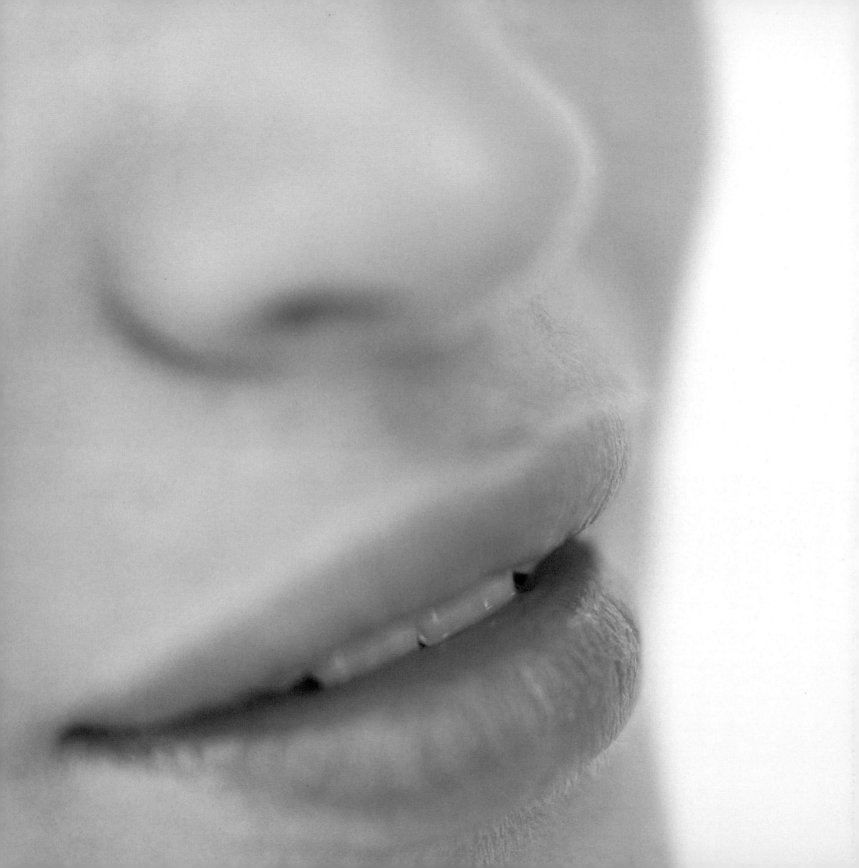

Self healing begins here…

The study of aromatherapy has largely been an ancedotal science. That means that much of the information about the therapeutic actions of essential oils has been compiled over the centuries by a process of trial and error. Thousands of aromatherapists and herbalists have researched and recorded their results concerning the actions of essential oils. Clinical investigations into the properties of particular oils are relatively recent, and in many cases have not been terribly thorough. The perfume and flavors industries have done quite a lot of research over the last decade or so, but the pharmaceutical industry is yet to do extensive research into the therapeutic actions of essential oils. These charts have been compiled by combining several of the best reference texts on essential oils written by qualified aromatherapists. This body of knowledge owes much to the experience and passion of aromatherapists who have diligently recorded their results with particular oils. Some of the oils mentioned in these charts are not covered in Chapter 3—The Good Oils.

Mind benders

When we talk about the science of aromatherapy, we are generally dealing with the direct chemical actions of the essential oils on the body. And when we speak of the art of aromatherapy, we are mostly concerned with the blending of essential oils to enhance moods, change emotional states, and pro-mote healing on subtle, energetic levels. Essential oils have the ability to alter mental and emotional states because they effect the hormones and the chemistry of the brain, as well as working on the more subtle energies of the body such as memory, feeling, and awareness. In this way essential oils are mood makers.

Most essential oils are suitable for baths, massage blends, and burning. Check the therapeutic actions of individual oils in Chapter 3 before prescribing them.

Choose one or more of these essential oils to revive or soothe your mental and emotional states:

Angry: bergamot, cedarwood, Roman chamomile, frankincense, lavender, lemon, myrrh, rose, sandalwood, ylang-ylang.

Anxious: basil, bergamot, geranium, lavender, neroli.

Balance: bergamot, clary sage, geranium, juniper, lavender, lemon, orange, rose, rosemary, sandalwood.

Concentration: basil, cedarwood, eucalyptus, juniper, lemon, neroli, orange, peppermint, rosemary, sandalwood, tea tree.

Confidence: bergamot, cedarwood, clary sage, frankincense, jasmine, neroli, rose.

Depression: bergamot, clary sage, patchouli, rose, ylang-ylang.

Euphoria: clary sage, jasmine, ylang-ylang.

Fears: bergamot, clary sage, geranium, marjoram, myrrh, neroli, orange, peppermint, rose, sandalwood, ylang-ylang.

Grief: bergamot, chamomile, clary sage, eucalyptus, frankincense, lavender, lemon, marjoram, orange, rose, sage, ylang-ylang.

Insomnia: bergamot, lavender, marjoram, neroli, orange.

Irritability: bergamot, cedarwood, clary sage, fennel, frankincense, grapefruit, juniper, lavender, lemon, lemongrass, neroli, rose, sandalwood.

Memory: basil, cinnamon, eucalyptus, fennel, lemon, pine, rosemary, sandalwood, tea tree.

Nervous butterflies: basil, bergamot, cedarwood, chamomile, geranium, lavender, neroli, rose.

Nightmares: bergamot, cedarwood, clary sage, eucalyptus, frankincense, marjoram, myrrh, neroli, rose, sage, sandalwood, ylang-ylang.

Obsessiveness: clary sage, geranium, lavender, marjoram, neroli, rose.

Resentment: rose.

Shock: chamomile, myrrh, neroli, ylang-ylang.

Stress: bergamot, lavender, neroli, patchouli, sandalwood.

Mood therapy

Use the following blends in vaporizers and burners, in baths or mixed in massage blends as mood therapy:

Balancing blend: geranium 4 drops, neroli 3 drops, rose 2 drops.

Calming blend: Roman chamomile 4 drops, rose 4 drops.

Euphoric blend: lavender 3 drops, orange 2 drops, clary sage 3 drops, ylang-ylang 2 drops.

Grounding blend: bergamot 3 drops, atlas cedar 2 drops, lavender 4 drops, sandalwood 3 drops.

Pampering blend: rose 3 drops, neroli 3 drops, lavender 3 drops.

Reviving blend: lemon 2 drops, peppermint 2 drops, pine 2 drops, rose 3 drops.

Uplifting blend: bergamot 4 drops, clary sage 3 drops, ylang-ylang 4 drops.

Physical therapy

Hippocrates said "the way to health is to have an aromatic bath and scented massage every day." The old guy was onto something. The combination of sweet smells, soothing massage, and potent oils produce thousands of chemical reactions that help balance the brain and body. Very few oils have just one action on the body—essential oils are extremely complex substances and can benefit the physiology in many ways. The following therapeutic index is a guide to using essential oils to safely treat some common ailments. Remember that essential oils should never replace the advice of a qualified physician, but they can bring relief and healing to many everyday problems.

Acne: benzoin, German chamomile, cedarwood, clove bud, geranium, juniper, lavender, neroli, orange, patchouli, rosemary, tea tree.

Air disinfectant: cypress, eucalyptus, grapefruit, juniper, lemon, orange, pine, sage.

Anti-aging: clary sage, frankincense, geranium, lavender, marjoram, neroli, orange, patchouli, rose otto, ylang-ylang.

Arthritis (rheumatoid): eucalyptus, German chamomile (inflammation), Roman chamomile, geranium, lemongrass.

Athlete's foot: bergamot, lavender, myrrh, peppermint, tea tree.

Bronchitis: cedarwood, clove bud, eucalyptus, frankincense, ginger, juniper, lavender, lemon, marjoram, myrrh, pine, rose otto, sage, tea tree, thyme.

Bruises: German chamomile, fennel, lemon, marjoram, myrrh, rosemary, sage.

Burns: benzoin, cedar, German chamomile, geranium, lavender, patchouli, sage.

Catarrh: cedarwood, lemon, marjoram, niaouli, peppermint, rosemary, sage.

Cellulite: cedarwood (lymphatic), geranium, lemongrass (circulation stimulant), patchouli (congestion), rosemary, sage (congestion), sandalwood (lymphatic).

Constipation: basil, fennel, ginger, juniper, mandarin, orange, rosemary.

Coughs and colds: cedarwood, cypress, eucalyptus, geranium, juniper, lavender, lemon, peppermint, pine, tea tree.

Cramps: basil, Roman chamomile (soothing), clary sage, fennel, lavender, marjoram, rosemary, sage.

Cuts/wounds: bergamot, cedarwood, German chamomile, clove bud (analgesic), cypress, frankincense, geranium (bleeding), lavender, myrrh, orange, patchouli, tea tree (infection).

Dermatitis: bergamot, German chamomile, eucalyptus (antibacterial), geranium, juniper, lavender, patchouli, rose otto, sage.

Diarrhea: Roman chamomile, cinnamon, clove bud, geranium, ginger, juniper, lemon, marjoram, peppermint, sandalwood.

Eczema: German chamomile (irritation), frankincense (weeping), geranium, lavender, patchouli (weeping), rose otto, sandalwood (weeping).

Flatulence: basil, bergamot, fennel, ginger, lavender, peppermint.

Flu: clove bud, eucalpytus, lavender, myrrh, peppermint, pine, rosemary, sage, tea tree.

Fluid retention: cedarwood, geranium (congestion), juniper, rosemary (congestion).

Fungal infections: clove, cypress, geranium, lavender, patchouli, peppermint, pine, rosemary, sage, sandalwood, thyme.

Gout: basil, Roman chamomile, fennel, grapefruit, juniper, pine, rosemary.

Headache: Roman chamomile, cypress, eucalyptus (congestive), lavender, lemon, peppermint (digestive), rosemary, sandalwood.

Heartburn: Roman chamomile, peppermint, sandalwood.

Herpes: bergamot, eucalyptus, geranium, lavender, lemon, sage.

High blood pressure: basil, juniper (diuretic), lavender, lemon, marjoram, ylang-ylang.

Impotence: cinnamon, ginger, peppermint, pine, rose otto, ylang-ylang.

Indigestion: basil (nervous), bergamot, fennel, ginger, lemon, lemongrass, mandarin, orange, peppermint, rosemary.

Inflammation: German and Roman chamomile, clary sage, frankincense, geranium, lavender, myrrh, rose otto, sandalwood.

Insect bites: basil, lavender, peppermint, sage, tea tree.

Insect repellent: basil, cedarwood, clove bud, eucalyptus, geranium, lavender, lemon, lemongrass, peppermint.

Insomnia: bergamot, Roman chamomile, cypress, geranium, lavender, lemon, mandarin, marjoram, melissa, neroli, orange, rose otto, sandalwood, ylang-ylang.

Irritation (skin): German and Roman chamomile, cedarwood, lavender, neroli, patchouli, rose.

Kidney (general): cedarwood, eucalyptus, fennel, geranium, juniper, lavender, lemon, pine, sage, sandalwood.

Liver (general): basil, Roman chamomile, juniper, lemon, lemongrass, peppermint, rosemary, thyme.

Low blood pressure: clove bud, grapefruit, neroli, rosemary, sage, thyme.

Menopause: Roman chamomile, clary sage, cypress, fennel, geranium, lemon, grapefuit, peppermint (hot flash), pine, rose otto, sage, sandalwood.

Menstruation (scanty): Roman chamomile, clary sage (hormonal), fennel, juniper, lavender, melissa (hormonal), rosemary, rose otto (hormonal).

Menstruation (painful): basil (congestion), clary sage, cypress (congestion), fennel, geranium, juniper, marjoram, peppermint, pine, sage (congestion).

Mental fatigue: basil, clove bud, peppermint, rosemary, sage.

Migraine: basil, German chamomile, eucalyptus, marjoram (menstrual), peppermint, rosemary.

Muscular pain: basil, camphor, German chamomile, frankincense, juniper, lavender, nutmeg (analgesic), rosemary, sage.

Nausea: fennel, ginger, mandarin (pregnancy), peppermint (travel), sandalwood (soothing).

Nervous exhaustion: basil (balancing), clary sage, clove bud, geranium, tea tree, thyme.

Neuralgia: Roman chamomile, clove bud, eucalyptus, juniper, lavender, peppermint, pine, rosemary, sandalwood.

Ovaries (general): clary sage (stimulant), cypress, rose, rosemary (regulator), sage, ylang-ylang (stimulant).

Palpitations: aniseed, basil, fennel, lavender, mandarin, melissa, neroli, petitgrain, rosemary, ylang-ylang.

Perspiration: basil, cypress, geranium, lavender, neroli, sage.

Premenstrual syndrome: Roman chamomile, clary sage, geranium, lavender, neroli, rose otto, sage (congestion), sandalwood.

Psoriasis: benzoin, bergamot, Roman chamomile, lavender, patchouli.

Respiratory infection: eucalyptus, frankincense, lemon, peppermint, petitgrain, pine (*see* bronchitis).

Rheumatism (muscular tightness): basil, clove bud, eucalyptus, frankincense, geranium (inflammation), ginger (warming), juniper, nutmeg (analgesic), rosemary (stiffness), sage, thyme.

Scars: cedarwood, frankincense, lavender, myrrh, patchouli.

Sciatica: Roman chamomile, clove bud, eucalyptus, juniper, lavender, peppermint, pine, rosemary, sandalwood.

Shingles: clove bud, eucalyptus, frankincense, geranium, peppermint, sage, tea tree.

Sinusitis: basil, clove bud, eucalyptus, marjoram, peppermint, pine, rosemary, sage, tea tree, thyme.

Skin (dry): German chamomile, Roman chamomile, geranium, lavender, neroli, petitgrain, damask rose, rose otto, sandalwood.

Skin (mature): benzoin, clary sage, fennel, frankincense, lavender, myrrh, neroli, rosemary, sandalwood.

Skin (oily): bergamot, cedarwood, cypress, geranium, juniper, lavender, lemon, rosemary, ylang-ylang.

Skin (sensitive): German and Roman chamomile, neroli, patchouli, rose otto.

Sore throat: cedarwood, clove bud, eucalyptus, geranium (inflammation), lavender, lemon, peppermint, sandalwood (soothing).

Sprains: lavender, marjoram, nutmeg (analgesic), rose, rosemary, sage.

Stress: bergamot, Roman chamomile, clary sage, fennel, lavender, marjoram, ylang-ylang.

Stretch marks: frankincense, geranium, lavender, myrrh, orange, patchouli.

Sunburn: geranium, lavender, sandalwood.

Tonic (circulation): rosemary (circulation), sage, sandalwood.

Tonic (muscles): (circulatory stimulants) clove, frankincense, marjoram, tea tree, thyme.

Toothache: Roman chamomile (teething), clove bud, pine, sage.

Travel sickness: ginger, peppermint.

Ulcers (skin): geranium, lavender, lemon, myrrh.

Vaginitis: German chamomile, lavender, tea tree (infection).

Varicose veins: basil, clary sage, juniper (stimulant), lemon, patchouli (decongestant), peppermint (cooling), rosemary (astringent), sandalwood (soothing).

Wrinkles: fennel, frankincense, myrrh, neroli, rose.

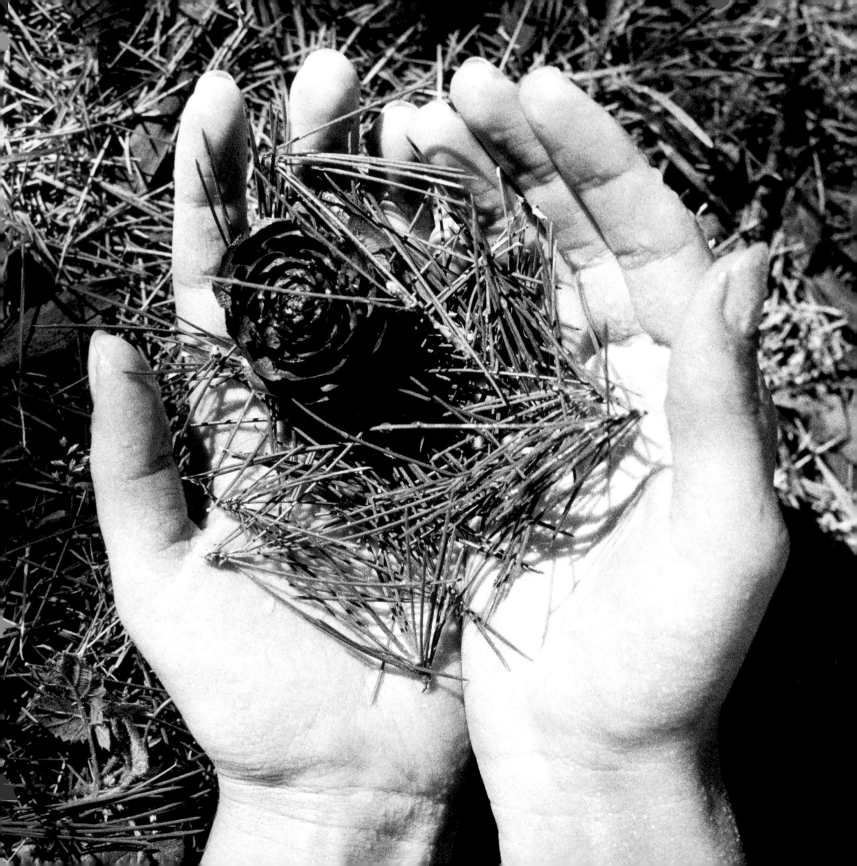

The following blends are suggested for some common ailments. But by all means, use your intuition to help you make blends to heal other minor health problems. These blends have been formulated as a guide and are calculated for ½ fl oz of carrier oil.

Arthritis and sore joints: *Massage* frankincense 3 drops, lavender 4 drops, lemongrass 2 drops.

Back pain: *Massage* lemongrass 3 drops, lavender 3 drops, peppermint 2 drops, sandalwood 1 drop.

Bronchitis: *Bath* eucalyptus 2 drops, juniper 3 drops, marjoram 2 drops, lavender 2 drops. *Inhalant* eucalyptus 4 drops, juniper 2 drops, marjoram 2 drops, rosemary 3 drops. *Massage* eucalpytus 4 drops, juniper 3 drops, marjoram 2 drops, rosemary 2 drops.

Chilblains: *Massage* lemon 4 drops, pine 3 drops, lavender 4 drops. *Foot and hand bath* lemon 3 drops, pine 2 drops, lavender 3 drops.

Head cold: *Massage* basil 3 drops, eucalyptus 3 drops, peppermint 2 drops. *Bath oil* basil 2 drops, eucalpytus 3 drops, lavender 4 drops. *Inhalant* basil 3 drops, eucalyptus 3 drops, peppermint 3 drops.

Cold with a cough: *Inhalant to remove mucus* bergamot 2 drops, sandalwood 2 drops, eucalyptus 3 drops, peppermint 1 drop. *Bath* lavender 3 drops, rosemary 3 drops.

Hangover: *Inhalant* rosemary 1 drop, lavender 3 drops, peppermint 2 drops. *Bath* juniper 3 drops, fennel 2 drops, rosemary 2 drops. *Cold compress* geranium 4 drops, lemon 2 drops.

Immune system: *Bath* bergamot 2 drops, rosemary 2 drops, eucalyptus 2 drops, geranium 2 drops, tea tree 2 drops. *Massage* bergamot 3 drops, lavender 4 drops, eucalyptus 2 drops, tea tree 2 drops.

Indigestion/heartburn: *Hot compress* bergamot 3 drops, peppermint 2 drops. *Massage* peppermint 2 drops, basil 2 drops, fennel 1 drop, orange 1 drop.

Insect repellent: *Massage* lemon 2 drops, geranium 2 drops, cedarwood 2 drops.

Insomnia: *Massage* bergamot 2 drops, Roman chamomile 3 drops, rose 3 drops. *Bath* orange 2 drops, lavender 2 drops, sandalwood 2 drops.

Irregular menstrual periods: *Massage* clary sage 3 drops, rose 3 drops, sandalwood 2 drops.

Menstrual pain: *Hot compress* clary sage 3 drops, marjoram 2 drops for abdomen and lower back. *Massage* sandalwood 3 drops, fennel 3 drops, geranium 3 drops. *Bath* sandalwood 3 drops, chamomile 3 drops, geranium 3 drops.

Migraine: *Bath* lavender 4 drops, marjoram 2 drops, rosemary 2 drops. *Massage head* basil 1 drop, peppermint 1 drop mixed with a teaspoon of jojoba oil and massaged into temples.

Muscular aches and pains: *Hot compress* chamomile 3 drops, rosemary 3 drops, frankincense 2 drops. *Massage* basil 2 drops, lavender 4 drops, rosemary 3 drops. *Bath* eucalyptus 2 drops, frankincense 2 drops, rosemary 2 drops.

Perspiration: *Massage* basil 2 drops, geranium 4 drops, cypress 2 drops. *Bath* lemon 3 drops, lavender 2 drops, neroli 2 drops.

Poor circulation: *Massage* lemon 3 drops, marjoram 3 drops, rosemary 4 drops. *Bath* lemon 3 drops, rosemary 2 drops, rose 2 drops.

Tonic for hair: *Massage* bergamot 2 drops, lavender 4 drops, chamomile 2 drops, cedarwood 2 drops.

Aromatherapist's recommended blends and expert advice

Ron Guba is a practicing aromatherapist and naturopath who has worked with essential oils and aromatherapy for more than twelve years. Ron is a dedicated scientist and extraordinary healer. His own company, Essential Therapeutics, distributes fine quality essential oils and cosmetic products. With the benefit of years of experience treating and healing hundreds of patients, his therapeutic aromatherapy blends have far-reaching benefits for the body, mind, and emotions. Blends are recommended for ½ fl oz of carrier oil.

Ron Guba's Skin Treatment Blends

Dry skin synergy: This blend is designed to stimulate proper functioning of the sebaceous glands, restoring balance to the skin.

Rose - 2 drops

Geranium - 2 drops

Lavender - 4 drops

Sandalwood - 2 drops

In a carrier of: Carrot oil, evening primrose oil, and sweet almond oil.

Oily combination-skin synergy: An effective treatment for overactive sebaceous glands, this blend will help treat and prevent acne.

Lavender - 1 drop

Bergamot - 1 drop

Rosemary - 1 drop

Lemon - 1 drop

Ylang-ylang - 1 drop

Atlas cedar - 1 drop

In a carrier of: Macadamia and avocado oil and jojoba.

Acne synergy: This blend will help reduce inflammation, clear blocked pores, control infection, and balance the activity of the sebaceous glands, calming acne-prone skin.

Neroli - 2 drops

Lavender - 2 drops

Geranium - 1 drop

Sage - 1 drop

Ylang-ylang - 1 drop

Sandalwood - 1 drop

In a carrier of: Evening primrose oil, sweet almond oil, and rose hip oil.

Couperose synergy: This blend is designed to strengthen and tone the capillaries, reducing sensitivity and redness.

Cypress - 2 drops

Rose - 2 drops

Lemon - 1 drop

Patchouli - 1 drop

German chamomile - 1 drop

In a carrier of: Avocado oil, evening primrose oil, and jojoba.

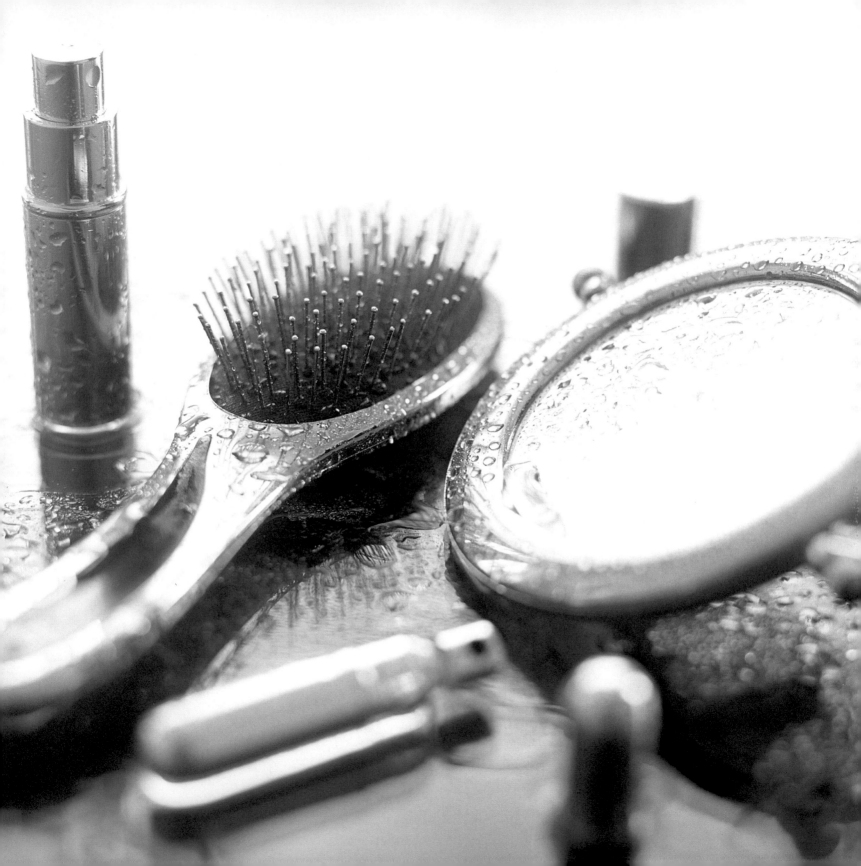

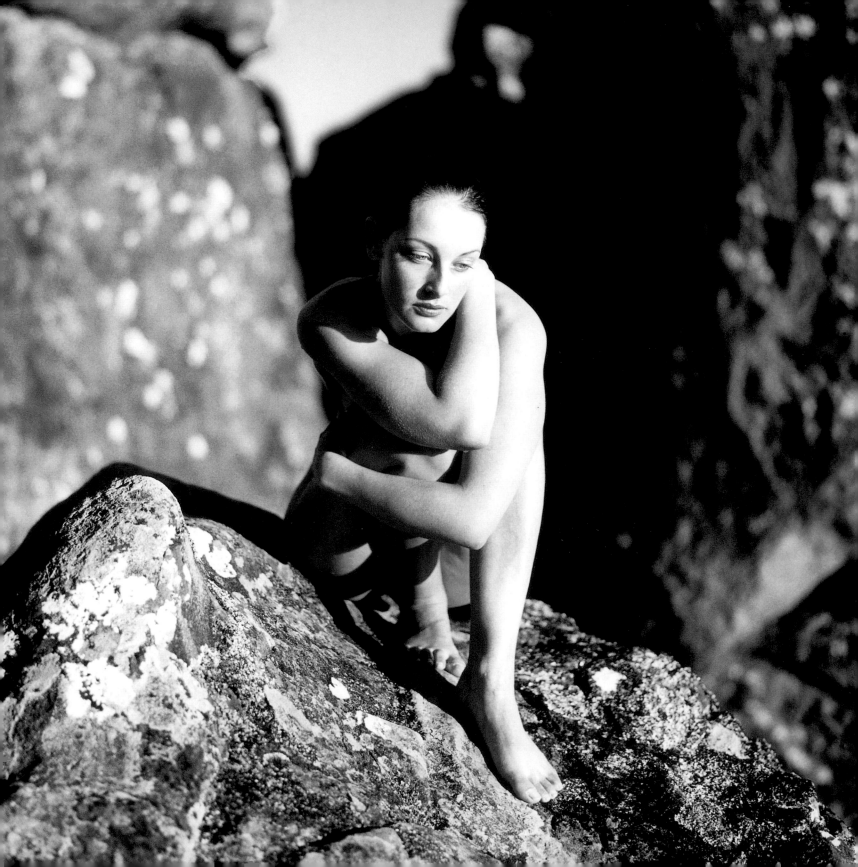

Dermatitis/sensitive skin synergy: This blend will help reduce the inflammation, irritation, and sensitivity associated with eczema, dermatitis, and other sensitive skin conditions.

German chamomile - 1 drop

Roman chamomile - 1 drop

Lavender - 4 drops

Clary sage - 1 drop

Patchouli - 2 drops

In a carrier of: Carrot oil, evening primrose oil, wheatgerm oil, and sweet almond oil.

Mature/devitalized skin synergy: A highly stimulating skin tonic, this blend will help boost cell turnover in the dermis and increase blood supply.

Lavender - 4 drops

Myrrh - 1 drop

Neroli - 2 drops

Rosemary - 1 drop

Rose - 1 drop

Sandalwood - 2 drops

In a carrier of: Carrot oil and avocado oil.

Monster kid blend: This blend will calm even the most mischievous children.

Lavender - 4 drops

Roman chamomile - 1 drop

Lemon - 1 drop

In a carrier of: Sweet almond oil for baths and massage.

Premenstrual blend: This blend is designed to help reduce the psychological and physiological signs and symptoms of premenstrual syndrome.

Rose - 2 drops

Roman chamomile - 1 drop

Geranium - 3 drops

Clary sage - 2 drops

In a carrier of: Sweet almond or grapeseed oil for massage (6–8 drops right into a bath).

Sooth my aching body blend: After a long hard day fighting it out on the corporate battlefield or playing hard in the sandpit, this blend will soothe aching muscles and relax the entire body.

Massage blend:

Basil - 2 drops

Lavender - 4 drops

Rosemary - 2 drops

Lemongrass - 1 drop

Clove bud - 1 drop

Bath blend:

Basil - 1 drop

Lavender - 3 drops

Rosemary - 1 drop

Marjoram - 1 drop

In a carrier of: Avocado oil and wheatgerm oil.

Laid-back blend: This blend will bring quiet to a busy brain, reducing mental and physical anxiety. Perfect before bed or those intimate moments when you want to be laid-back, cool, calm, and collected.

Roman chamomile - 1 drop

Lavender - 2 drops

Bergamot - 2 drops

Sandalwood - 1 drop

In a carrier of: Grapeseed oil, and dropped into the bath or massaged into the shoulders, neck, and back.

Rejuvenating Blend: Boosting the immune system as well as bringing clarity to the mind, this blend is great for an instant pick-me-up or long-term rejuvenation.

Eucalyptus - 2 drops

Tea tree - 2 drops

Geranium - 2 drops

Sage - 1 drop

In a carrier of: Evening primrose oil and grapeseed oil for baths and massage.

Ready willing and able blend: For those times when you want to take on the world and feel a surge of personal power. This blend will boost your confidence, enhancing your ability to focus and make decisions on your feet.

Orange - 2 drops

Lavender - 3 drops

Frankincense - 1 drop

Grapefruit - 1 drop

In a carrier of: Grapeseed oil and wheatgerm oil for baths and massage.

Woe is me blend: When the world starts getting you down, this blend provides a helping hand when you need it most reviving flagging energies and kick-starting the entire system.

Rose - 1 drop

Jasmine - 1 drop

Orange - 3 drops

Bergamot - 2 drops

In a carrier of: Avocado oil for baths and massage.

Night owl's salvation blend: The insomniac's rescue remedy, this blend will help you sleep like a baby.

Roman chamomile - 1 drop

Bergamot - 3 drops

Marjoram - 2 drops

Lemon - 1 drop

In a carrier of: Grapeseed oil for baths and massage. Dropped onto the pillow at night or sprinkled onto a tissue.

Traveler's best friend blend: Every traveler knows the perils of traveling without a fully equipped medicine kit. This blend is the perfect companion for adventurers, a trusty cure-all for those icky, sticky, smelly, nasty things you can pick up on the road to nirvana.

Lavender - 2 drops

Tea tree - 2 drops

Peppermint - 1 drop

Basil - 1 drop

In a carrier of: Grapeseed oil and wheatgerm oil for baths. Use tea tree as a general topical antiseptic.

Red hot lover blend: Love potions may not be the stock-in-trade of modern perfumers, but in the seventeenth century, France and Italy provided the industry with handsome returns. This blend has aphrodisiac properties that can melt the hardest of hearts and excite the most dormant hormones into unfamiliar flights of fancy.

Neroli - 1 drop

Rose - 1 drop

Ylang-ylang - 1 drop

Orange - 2 drops

Bergmot - 3 drops

Patchouli - 1 drop

In a carrier of: Avocado oil and evening primrose oil for baths and massage.

Stressed out employee blend: When you're overworked, overtired, and oversensitive, this blend is designed to help bring focus to overspent minds and calm overwrought nerves.

Rosemary - 2 drops

Roman chamomile - 1 drop

Geranium - 1 drop

Lemon - 2 drops

Sandalwood - 1 drop

In a carrier of: Sweet almond oil or evening primrose oil for baths and massage. Drop this mixture into a burner on the desk in your office.

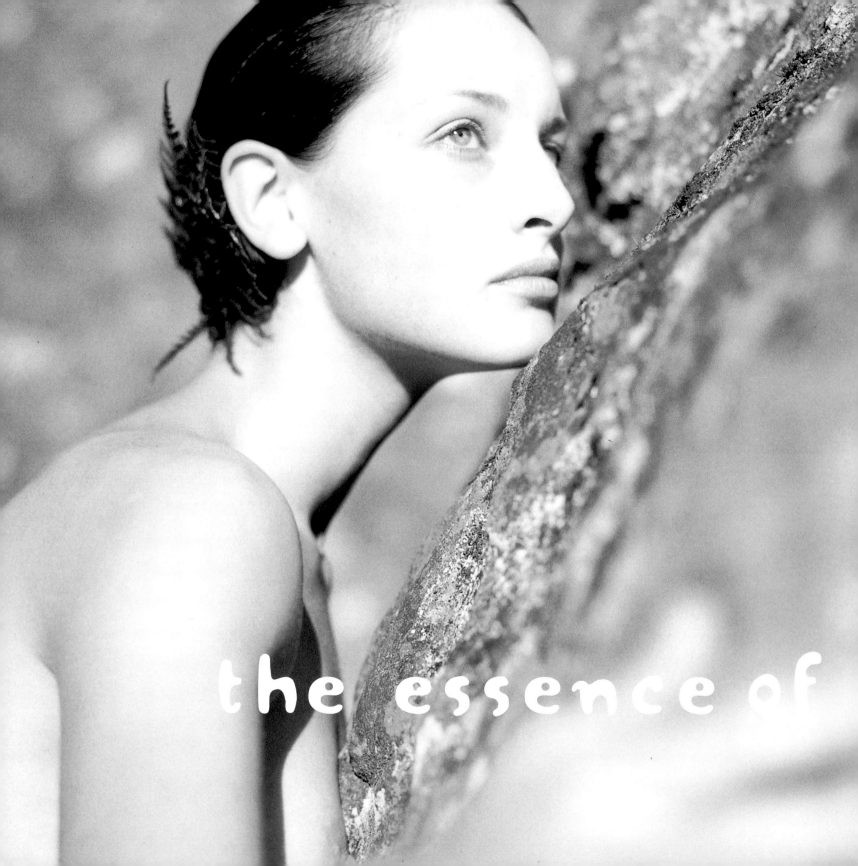

the essence of

The
central premise of
all alternative therapies,
including aromatherapy, is
the notion that in order to heal
and maintain health, the practitioner
must treat the whole organism—mind, emotions, body,
and spirit. In aromatherapy, the idea is to use natural substances
to activate the body's own healing mechanisms. Unlike drugs,
essential oils are complete, complex biological entities, which is the
reason they have holistic healing benefits for the body. The oils themselves
are amazing natural medicines and will treat the body effectively, but
what's really important about aromatherapy is that it embraces a shift in
thinking about how we treat and heal the body. This philosophy takes into
account the natural world and aims to preserve the environment. This
philosophy wants to help the body help itself and is searching for the reasons
why we get sick, not simply treating the symptoms. It also enables us to
touch and pamper ourselves in the process of healing. Currently,
medicine is searching for ways to encourage the body to heal
itself. Researchers are investigating the role of the immune
system in fighting disease and are looking for new therapies
and drugs that will stimulate the body's own
immune response. Aromatherapy is at the
front line of twenty-first-century
medicine.

health

A guide to life-long balance and bliss

We
all know that,
because viruses and
bacteria have quickly
evolved resistant strains
to pharmaceuticals, our
reliance on antibiotics is
fast coming to a close.
Preventive health
care from childhood
throughout adult
life is becoming
vital to human
survival.

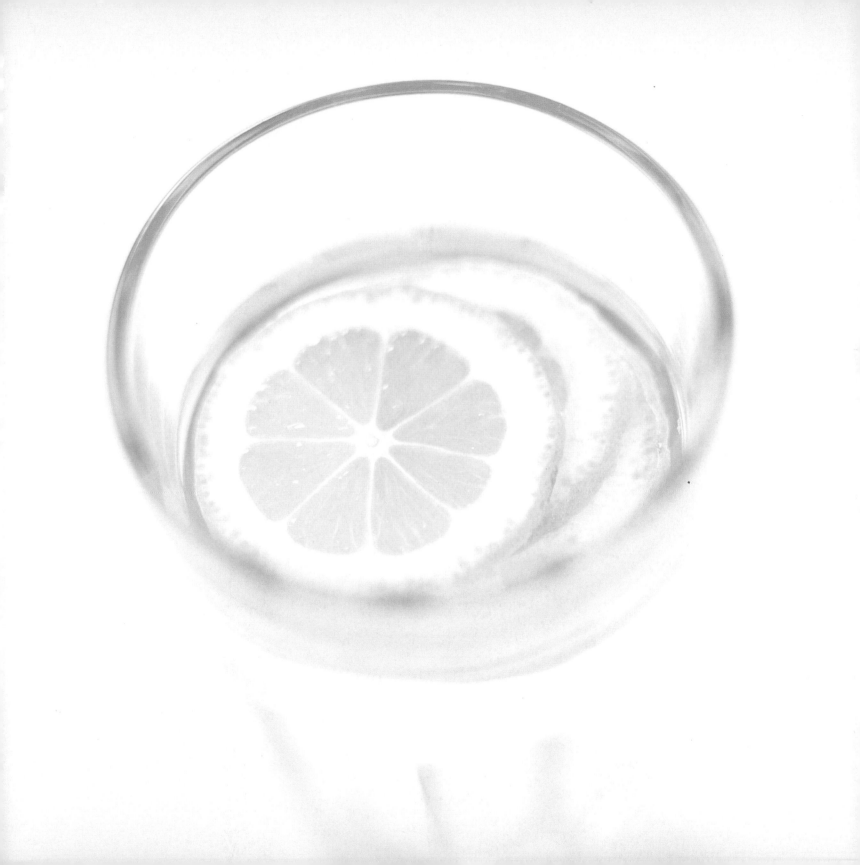

The human immune system

Since the beginning of time, humans have searched for ways to protect and enhance life. Although nature designed humans to live a limited time on Earth, creating sickness and disease to keep numbers in check, she also gave humans a fully equipped arsenal to give each and every individual a fighting chance of survival on the planet.

The human immune system is principally responsible for fighting off disease, and part of its role is to manufacture antibodies to target specific aggressors. The immune system also works closely with other systems of the body, including the endocrine system, the internal organs, the brain, and the skin—which itself is actually part of the immune system. When the immune system is depressed, or not working properly, the body's guard system is down, giving illness a chance to take over the body. On a simple level, it's obvious that when we are tired and run-down we are more susceptible to colds and flu. Stress, poor diet, lack of exercise, lack of stimulation, lack of touch, and pollution all take their toll on the immune system.

Many things are known to stimulate the immune system, including general well-being and happiness, good nutrition, touch, pleasant smells, exercise, and meditation. This incredibly sophisticated system acts as an internal healer, constantly bringing the body back into balance and health.

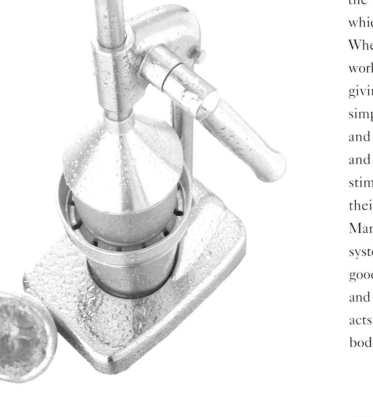

154

Essential oils and the immune system

Essential oils have an amazing affinity with the human immune system. They stimulate the secretion of immunoglobulins, which produce antibodies to help fight infection and disease. The antibacterial, antimicrobial, anti-inflammatory, antiviral, and immunostimulant properties of plants can help the body at every level of biological functioning. The mere smell of an essential oil is enough to send endorphins rushing to the brain, shooting messages of well-being throughout the entire body. Massaging the skin stimulates the immune system, and when essential oils are used, they help promote the effectiveness of all the body's defense systems.

Essential oils work by helping the body help itself, but they can't do it alone. Aromatherapy can achieve extraordinary results as a form of preventive medicine, but it would be foolish to hope that essential oils will cure all our problems—it's almost the same as going to the doctor and asking for a pill to fix everything from a broken heart to a broken leg.

Healing is an active process and cannot occur unless the patient becomes involved in his or her own well-being. If human beings are to live long, productive lives they need to take responsibility for their health and learn to implement basic wellness strategies such as good nutrition, regular exercise, rest, and meditation. This chapter is not designed to teach nutrition, meditation, and exercise; it is merely a guide to good living. The guidelines here will help support a fully functioning immune system, but they should not replace the advice of a health care professional trained in nutrition, exercise, or meditation.

Diet and your well-being

Nutrition is the basis of good health. Many of the diseases present in our society are preventable and can be addressed with basic nutrition and common sense. The body is a complex and sophisticated piece of biochemical machinery. It needs the right fuel in order to run efficiently. Food provides the body with energy, and low energy levels are often an indicator of poor health. Many illnesses such as arthritis, cancer, and heart disease; infections such as cystitis and irritable bowel syndrome; dermatitis, digestive disorders, headaches, mental illnesses, eczema, asthma, PMS, and high blood pressure are attributable to poor nutrition.

It is important, therefore, to eat a diet rich in foods that will stimulate the immune system—foods that contain "life-generating" forces such as sprouted seeds and grains, fresh fruit and raw vegetable juices. These foods have active healing properties and assist rapid biological transformations. A diet designed to boost energy will also consist of fresh, unprocessed whole vegetables, nuts, fruits, and raw dairy products, such as goat's milk and yogurt. Cooked vegetables, grains, and animal proteins such as fish, chicken, and meat should constitute a smaller part of the diet. Canned foods, processed foods, and refined foods that contain white sugar and white flour should represent the smallest part of the diet. Excessive fat or sugar intake contributes to the accumulation of wastes in the tissues and can impair proper cellular metabolism.

By removing or restricting the intake of refined and highly processed foods, foods that are often the causes of allergies and sensitivities, the body has a chance to carry out elimination normally—reducing the risk of disease, lethargy, and poor health.

It stands to reason that when people are put on diets high in fresh, whole foods they suddenly glow—they feel lighter, more energetic, and optimistic about life.

Exercise and your health

Exercise is essential for the continued well-being of both body and mind. Physiologically, we need exercise to maintain a healthy, properly functioning body and immune system. On the mental level, exercise has many benefits. Recent research reveals that physical activity triggers the release of natural, pleasure-boosting chemicals from the brain. These endorphins and encephalins are natural pain-killers and are produced by both physical and mental processes, but in particular strenuous exercise. These chemicals are part of the functioning of the immune system, keeping disease and depression at bay.

The body needs regular and varied exercise in order to keep muscles, joints, ligaments, and tendons strong and supple. A regular walk will produce all the chemical reactions necessary for maintaining a reasonably fit body, but the walk itself can also be a pleasurable life-enhancing experience. Breathing in fresh air, taking in the beauty of nature, enjoying the company of a friend, or perhaps the "moving meditation" of letting the thoughts and stresses of life dissolve with the pleasure of exercise, are all part of living well. Exercise helps us embrace life. When we feel strong, fit, and healthy, we are better equipped to fight disease and take the stresses and strains of modern life. A seventy-year-old jogger is more likely to have a healthy immune system than a forty-five-year-old couch potato. Part of the reason is the simple mechanics of keeping the body in good working order, but the other important factor is that the seventy-year-old is dancing with the rhythm of life. Age can be a state of mind as well as body, and regular exercise will help you believe you are fit, young, and strong.

Meditation and your well-being

Meditation aims to remove the outside distractions of everyday life, allowing the meditator to quietly retreat inside and search for peace and harmony. Regular practitioners report improvements not only in their health but in their emotional and psychological states as well. Meditation has been used to achieve deep states of relaxation and altered states of consciousness for many thousands of years. There are many forms of meditation, most of which originate in the East—India, China, and Japan—but the Native Americans and the Australian Aborigines also have their own meditation practices, which are mostly used to achieve higher states of awareness

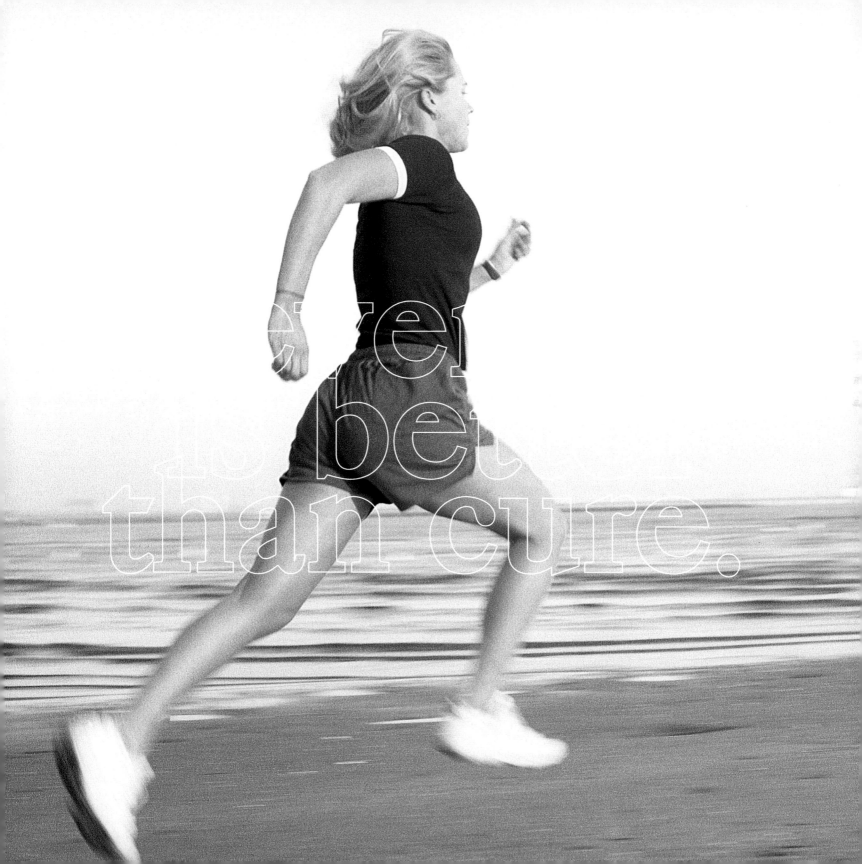

and are practiced as part of ritual ceremonies.

Meditation is one easy way to keep stress at bay. The effects are cumulative, which means that over a period of time, meditators discover that their lives improve. Traffic jams don't seem to bother them so much, their creativity levels rise, their energy for life increases, their relationships become more har-monious, and their intuition becomes sharper.

Meditation is a pathway to the unconscious. It's a tool that enables us to plumb the depths of the soul and discover the true nature of life—right at its harmonious, happy, loving source. Meditation masters say that the practice helps us get in touch with the universal energy that underlies all life, a vast ocean of bliss that breathes love into every creature, plant, person, and planet in the universe. By staring into a candle flame, repeating a mantra (sacred sound), or by simply concentrating on the breath, meditators can unlock the secrets of health and well-being.

The mind and body are one

More than 300 years ago, the philosopher Descartes theorized that the universe and all things within it were automated like a gigantic machine. From Descartes' time to the beginning of this century, science set out specifically to discover how the great machine worked. For the last 300 years we have looked at the mechanics of the natural world, the human body, and the universe. Today many of the theories that governed the way science approached its conclusions are being dispelled. Quantum physics has already begun to reshape the way we view ourselves and the universe, and as the ideas and experiments of this cutting edge science percolate down into the mainstream, it will become more and more obvious that many of the paradigms we have commonly accepted about the body and universe will no longer apply.

Traditionally, Western medicine has viewed the human body in a mechanistic way. We have looked at the body as a car that breaks down, in terms of working parts that could be replaced if they faltered or targeted with drugs when something goes wrong. Allopathic, or Western, medicine has looked at the symptoms and devised a cure through a process of deduction. It's a highly technical and specialized form of science. Doctors even divide the body into its component parts and specialize in that area of medicine. For example, neurologists deal with the brain, cardiologists deal with the heart, and immunologists concern themselves with the immune system.

When we are sick we go to the doctor to get fixed, like a car goes to an auto body shop after a crash. If the family doctor can't work out the problem, he or she will send you to a specialist, who will apply all of his or her specialist skills to treat the condi-tion. There is no question that this system of med-icine has been highly effective in treating many of the diseases that afflict humanity, but it has over-looked one very important part of healing. The body is a whole organism: The stomach does not get sick without the arms, the skin, the brain, and the immune system knowing about it. Although we may get better by treating the stomach upset in isolation, we have not explored the reason for the illness, nor the side effects of treating the stomach without taking into account the rest of the body.

Healthy mind, healthy body may be a time-honored aphorism, but it's only recently that the truth behind it, the connection between the mind and body, has become the focus of exploration by Western medicine.

A series of experiments performed in the 1970s isolated minute chemicals called neurotransmit-ters, which are used by the nervous system to transmit information—including thought process-es—throughout the body. Scientists were excited to find that these neurotransmitters existed well beyond the physical boundaries of the brain. The researchers also found evidence that a neurotrans-mitter called impramine, which is produced in abnormal quantities in the brains of clinically de-pressed people, had turned up in skin cells. The implication of that discovery was that depressed people not only have sad brains but sad skin, livers, lungs, and other organs, thanks to the presence of impramine throughout the body.

Similar studies revealed that neurotransmitters associated with stress could be found not only in the adrenal glands of anxiety sufferers but in their blood as well. Thanks to this new physical evidence, Western medicine is beginning to appreciate the fact that the health of the mind has a direct bearing on the well-being of the whole body. Of course, these Western researchers are only confirming what Eastern medical practitioners have known all along (even Hippocrates counseled his medical students to take account of their patients' emotions when looking at their ailments, but the notion somehow became all but lost in the evolution of Western medicine).

Based in the United States, Dr. Deepak Chopra is one of the leading exponents of using the power of the mind to heal the body. His beliefs are based on what he calls "Quantum Healing" (also the name of his best-selling book). It's a theory that suggests everything in the universe, including the energy humans generate in their own minds, is intercon-nected. Dr. Chopra believes his mission in life is to teach humans how to unlock the quantum energy in their minds that can be put to use to heal disease. To that end, he spends much of his time on the international lecture circuit. He says, "The hardest thing to get people to understand is how to use the power of the mind. As a concept it's difficult to grasp that the mind is not located in the brain, not just in the body, but is the fabric of the entire universe. Harnessing this great power is the medicine of the future."

In his book *Quantum Healing* Dr. Chopra explains, "We could say that the brain and the immune system are not like each other—they are each other, because they operate within the same chemical network. This means that to be happy and fight disease is much the same thing at a molecular level."

It has been said that the body is a perfect natural apothecary. The aim of all these complex studies is to better understand and more frequently employ the body's natural healing powers that can be prompted by the brain and behavior. American neuropharmacologist Candace Pert, Ph.D., says, "On some level people possess within themselves the drug to cure every ill."

It sounds mind-boggling, but for the purposes of this book it is sufficient to understand that the old ways of treating illness—by isolating the symptoms and simply treating them without regard for the mind and emotions—is a clumsy way to treat the complexity of the human organism. Medicine must address the whole person and the environment in which that person lives. Medicine must also come to terms with the concept that healing is a dynamic process that involves an energy much greater than the body. When we heal ourselves, we come in contact with the quantum field, the universal mind—the level of energy where all life, all ideas, all magic, and miracles begin and end.

To conclude...

As a holistic practice, aromatherapy teaches you to look after every part of yourself—your body, mind, emotions, and spirit. This concept of holism is perhaps the most important part of aromatherapy. When you help your body help itself—by treating it with good food, plenty of rest, regular exercise, and pampering it with essential oils—it will respond in miraculous ways.

Humans have always looked to the plant world for remedies to ill health, and essential oils are perhaps the most accessible medicines available to modern people. However, let's not forget the role of the mind and emotions in the healing process. Some-where locked within every human being is the power to be well and happy, but the stresses of modern life often rob us of this innate knowledge. In the hustle and bustle we forget that we can help ourselves and too often run to the doctor for a prescription. Aromatherapy is a catalyst to good health because it *reminds* us that we can heal ourselves.

Transported on the fragrance of the floral world, we are sent into the deep recesses of our own brains and immune systems where the information we need to heal ourselves is stored. Aromatherapy links us to our primitive origins. It reminds us of a time when we were in harmony with the entire planet, when we understood the relationship between all things. The smells of essential oils excite in us an immediate healing—a connection to nature, a connection to our own wild nature, the medicine man, the shaman, the alchemist, the witch doctor within us all.

Further Reading

Aromatherapy: An A–Z
by Patricia Davis
Published by C W Daniel

The Practice of Aromatherapy
by Jean Valnet
Published by Inner Tradition

Magical Aromatherapy
by Scott Cunningham
Published by Llewellyn

Aromatherapy Workbook
by Shirley Price
Published by Thorsons

Practical Aromatherapy
by Shirley Price
Published by Thorsons

*The Dancing Wu Li Masters:
An Overview of the New Physics*
by Gary Zukav
Published by Bantam

Aromatherapy
by Viktor Blevi and Gretchen Sween
Published by Avon

A Natural History of Senses
by Diane Ackerman
Published by Random House

Quantum Healing
by Deepak Chopra
Published by Bantam

Ageless Body, Timeless Mind
by Deepak Chopra
Published by Crown

Jitterbug Perfume
by Tom Robbins
Published by Bantam

How to Get Well
by Paavo Airola, Ph.D.
Published by Health Plus

*Perfumery:
The Psychology & Biology of Fragrance*
edited by Steve Van Toller and George H. Dodd
Published by Chapman & Hall

Perfume
by Patrick Suskind
translated by John E. Woods
Published by Viking Penguin

Fragrance: The Story of Perfume from Cleopatra to Chanel
by Edwin T. Morris
Published by Scribner's Sons New York

Infant Massage: A Handbook for Loving Parents
by Vimala Schneider
Published by Bantam

The First Love Stories
by Diane Wolkstein
Published by HarperCollins

Essential Oils in the Body
by Tony Balacs
Published by Aromatherapy Publications

The Immune System of Mankind
by Dr. Daniel Penoel
Published by Aromatherapy Publications

Index

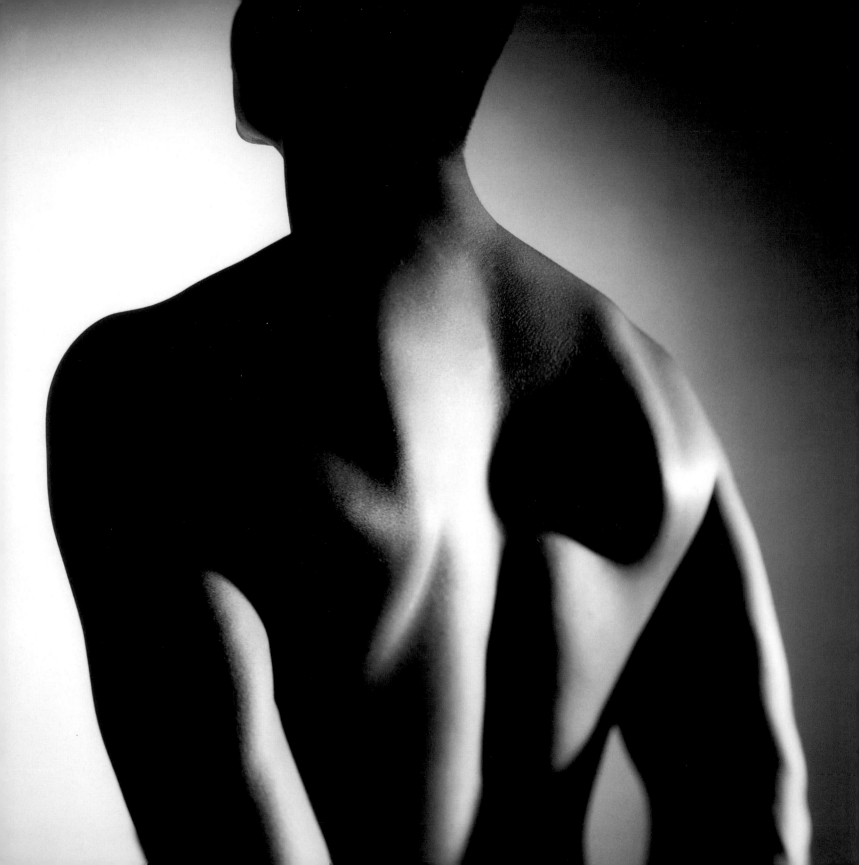

Acknowledgments

All my thanks must go to Andrew Hoyne and Rob Blackburn, my talented partners in this book. Their inspiration, support, dedication, and incredible ability has made this project a joy from start to finish.

Many thanks and appreciation to Ron Guba for sharing his wealth of knowledge so generously with me and whose scientific genius, humility, and wisdom helped me enormously.

Special thanks to Geoffrey Kempler for his continued support, energy, and enthusiasm.

Many thanks to Lisa Green for her sensitive editing.

Thanks to Deborah McLean who kept this project together and who lent her enormous talents so generously.

My thanks to David Wehner who gave his support and wisdom to this book.

Jane Burridge and Alison Urqhart deserve a special thanks for holding my hand and being the most fabulous agents in town.

Many thanks to everybody in Andrew's studio who gave energy, clarity, and enthusiasm.

My love and appreciation to my friends who have always encouraged me: Georgie Rogers, Darienne Sutton, Romaine Youdale, Harvey Collis, Melissa Caplice, Sophie Toomey, Amanda Clarke, Elaine Briggs, Tom Curtis, Alix Johnson, Lisa Vugich, Laura Courtney, Arkie Whiteley, Laura Boomer, Peter and Suzanne Noble, Trish Ruwald, Beverley Corlette, Robbie Anderson, Robyn Fowler-Smith, Nichola Kelly, Kerry Redgate, Penelope Ward, Steve Paridis, Amanda Adare, the Jacob family, Jacqueline Pittman, Melinda Screen, Antony Whitaker, Simon Rogers, Gen and Em Sharma, Professor Shan, Shona Barker, Siddhi and Sally Phillips.

Susan Irvine deserves a very special thanks for all her encouragement, love, and inspiration.

Last but not least I would like to thank my family, Sue, Joe, Georgie, and Andrew for being the warm, wonderful, exraordinary people that they are.

Dedicated

To Rowan for your constant love, support, tolerance, compassion, patience, and understanding throughout this process.

Nikki Goldstein

Firstly, my thanks go to Nikki and Rob for having faith in this project, in me, and that I could make it happen. You're both true professionals and extraordinarily talented to boot. You both are what others dream to be. Together we've made this book happen.

Thanks to everybody in my studio. You guys watch me invent these projects that seem far fetched, but you always get excited and encourage me. Your enthusiasm is my fuel.

Special thanks go to Linda Petrone for her extra support, and who's seen this project from start to finish.

Thanks also go to Anna Svigos and Angela Ho for their assistance in the important, difficult, and laborious job of typesetting this book.

Much appreciation and thanks to Deb McLean. Your enthusiasm should be bottled and sold at a premium. Thanks for all your help.

Thanks to Geoffrey at Aveda for introducing me to Nikki. Huge thanks to Andrea at Kleins Perfumery in Melbourne. Thanks to Greg Tyshing at Giant Model Management for helping us with some of the models. Thanks to Sally Bailey. Thanks to Jane Timberlake. Thanks to Sue Hines for her encouragement and knowledge. Thanks to Judy in Apollo Bay for letting us photograph her herb gardens. Thanks to Vanessa, Foong Ling, and Lynn. Thanks to EGO in Melbourne for great scans.

To all my favorite bars and restaurants, and Acland Street in general. Thanks to all my good friends and anybody who's been optimistic and had faith that we could crack the overseas publishing market.

Thanks to Warner Books' people: Mari Okuda, Maura Gibbons, Milton Batalion, Amye Dyer, Karen Casiano, and Suzanne Abel. Thanks to Jackie Merri Meyer for publishing this book. We had no shortage of offers, but Jackie had true passion and I know we'll do great things together.

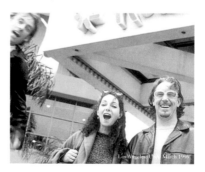

Los Angeles USA March 1996

Special thanks to Stef for her encouragement and love.

See you in the next book.

Andy Hoyne
ahoyne@c031.aone.net.au

Many thanks to Andrea at Kleins for the beautiful objects she made available to us. Thanks to our models Vicki, Kimberley, Rachelle, Cecily, Rebecca, Ari, Brad, Sally, Rachel, Neil, Kathryn, and baby Peppa, who is now out in the world and a joy to behold. Thank you Vivien Ashworth and Michelle Cutelli for beautiul makeup and hair. Eternal gratitude to Deb McLean—we would never have made it without you. Olivia, thank you for patience, advice, and encouragement. And of course, thank you Nikki and Andrew, you guys are the best!

Rob Blackburn

The beauty
of aromatherapy
is that you don't have to
have a degree in biochemistry,
a Ph.D. in psychology, or a master's
in massage to apply the principles
of this transformational art and
science to yourself, your
friends, and your
family.